Managing a Hospital Turnaround:

From crisis to profitability in three challenging years

Michael E. Rindler

Pluribus Press, Chicago

Library of Congress Catalog Card Number:
87-61937

International Standard Book Number:
0-931028-95-7

Pluribus Press, Inc.
160 East Illinois Street
Chicago, Illinois 60611

91 90 89 88   5 4 3 2

Printed in the United States of America

ibus Press, Inc.
erved

ress Catalog Card Number:

andard Book Number:

, Inc.
Street
60611

5 4 3 2

United States of America

Managing

From
in thr

M

Plurib

Library of Co
87-61937

International
0-931028-95-

Pluribus Pr
160 East Illin
Chicago, Illin

91   90   89

Printed in th

To the employees
of Beloit Memorial Hospital

Contents

Foreword

A 1987 REPORT from the American Hospital Association's Data Center said 414 hospitals had closed during the preceding five years. The number of closures had declined during the first two years of that period, and then increased in each of the succeeding years—by 36 percent 1986 over 1985. The majority of institutions that closed were small community hospitals whose average size was 68 beds, and most of them were located in rural areas, the report said. A publication by Touche Ross & Co., accountants, added a somber footnote: The majority of respondents to a Touche Ross survey of hospital executives in 1986 said they believed five to ten percent of U.S. hospitals would fail within the next five years, and 43 percent said they felt their own hospitals were "vulnerable to failure."

Given that the phrase is obviously so imprecise that it might be argued that 100 percent of hospitals are vulnerable to failure, these reports from A.H.A. and Touche Ross are nevertheless formidable enough to suggest that even the most optimistic and confident of hospital executives would be well advised to read this report of how one institution was turned back from the brink of disaster. This book is not only a road map of the way back to fiscal and professional well-being; for the institution that is already there, it offers a catalogue of policies and programs to make certain things will get better instead of worse.

Besides, Rindler is a masterly storyteller. To be sure, he did not create the story here as an artist would create a landscape. The characters in his story are the people who were there; these events happened and are in the minutes and reports of the hospital. Rindler's account is not a creation but a recording. The frankness and artlessness with which he tells about the triumphs in which he played the leading role are thus as disarming as his accounting of the times when his performance fell short or missed a critical turn in the road.

Either way, it's all spelled out here, and if the estimates reported by Touche Ross and A.H.A. are anywhere near right, the situation that Rindler found when he got to Beloit is going to be duplicated again and again in the years ahead. Unquestionably, Rindler himself will play the reprise of the Beloit story—perhaps more than once; these scenarios do not go unremarked in a profession that has many of the characteristics of a fraternity. Others who find themselves in the same kind of situation can be thankful if they have boards of trustees as understanding and as willing to keep their hands and noses out of operations as Rindler's trustees were.

Here it is then, unvarnished, from the day Rindler got to town and took over at the depleted and demoralized hospital, through the painful firings and layoffs, up to and through the decisions to add new services and make new alliances. For anyone taking over a failing hospital this account is a directory listing the things that have to be done—things that for the most part are difficult and unpleasant to do. To his credit, Rindler never stayed out of sight and let his assistants and department heads take the hard ones. He was out front all the time following his rule for the chief executive: "See and be seen."

In a city of 40,000 or so whose hospital is one of the major employers, it isn't much fun to be the person held responsible for wholesale layoffs; for months, Rindler was the town's leading pariah, and it wasn't long before the ranks of his detractors were joined by some of the community's leading citizens—the doctors at his own hospital, who were offended when he saw a need for recruiting new and improved talent for specialties like cardiology, outpatient services and a few other departments generally considered to be medicine's inviolable precincts.

It should be pointed out, however, that the lessons here aren't for only the beleaguered. The thoughtful reader whose problems are still on the far horizon will find in this turnaround experience a rich store of strategies that can be as useful to safeguard assets and meet competition as they were to Rindler in rescuing an institution on the brink. Either way, the lucky ones will be those who have read his book.

—Robert M. Cunningham Jr.
September, 1987

You Know You Are in Trouble When...

THIS BOOK is for hospitals facing financial troubles. That is a wide audience these days. The need for improved cost and quality control confronts virtually all healthcare institutions. This need won't diminish for a long time. The strategies described here are applicable in any hospital setting. Common sense and a passion for quality are the key ingredients in a hospital turnaround. The ability to keep smiling while being attacked from all sides and absolute fearlessness in dealing with physicians come in handy too. Turnarounds are not for executives with faint hearts and weak stomachs.

How does a hospital know it needs to be turned around? An affirmative answer to any of these warning sign questions is enough to conclude your hospital is in trouble.

1. Has the hospital operated at a loss on operations for two or more consecutive years?

2. Are activity trends significantly worse than those in competing hospitals?

3. Are trustees holding private meetings to discuss "concerns" or hiring outside management consultants to evaluate the chief executive officer's performance?

4. Has market share declined for two or more consecutive years?

5. Is the hospital always responding to marketing initiatives of competing hospitals, rather than the other way around?

6. Are physicians controlling policy decisions because of a weak board and management?

7. Are competing hospitals or a hospital chain offering to buy or merge with the hospital?

8. Are the hospital's bankers expressing concern about the ability to cover fixed expenses like interest on outstanding loans?

If the answer to any of these questions is "yes" for your hospital, update your résumé or get going to resolve the problems.

The turnaround of Beloit Memorial Hospital is the subject of this book. The hospital was in big trouble. Its turnaround is a tribute to the dedicated efforts of its board, management, physicians and employees. Beloit Memorial Hospital is a community not-for-profit hospital opened in 1970. At the time the turnaround began in 1984, it operated 180 beds and employed a staff of 700. The medical staff consisted of 45 physicians. Beloit is a typical midwest small city of 40,000 residents. There are five competing hospitals within twenty miles of Beloit. All were better managed and enjoyed better reputations than Beloit Memorial Hospital.

Beloit Memorial Hospital's activity and financial trends for the six year period 1978 through 1984 confirmed that the hospital was headed for disaster. Inpatient census had dropped 41 percent, from an average of 170 to an average of 100. Beloit's loss of inpatient business was substantially greater than that of hospitals in Wisconsin and throughout the nation. Activity declines accelerated to the crisis point in 1983-1984. That year 28 percent of its inpatient business was lost. At the time of these precipitous declines, the population of the greater Beloit community grew slightly. Unem-

FIGURE 1

1983-1984 Activity Trends

PATIENT DAY DECLINES
1983-1984

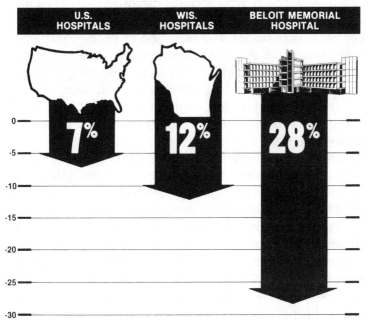

ployment declined slightly, from 12 percent to 10 percent.
Figure 1 illustrates how Beloit's 1983-1984 performance
compared with other U.S. and Wisconsin hospitals.

While the hospital's activity was declining, its financial
condition also deteriorated. The hospital lost approximately
$1.5 million between 1978 and 1983. It had lost another
$1.0 million between 1970 and 1977, bringing its cumula-
tive losses to $2.5 million since opening. It was projected to
lose an additional $500,000 in 1984. Poor profitability oc-

curred in spite of implementing, on average, an eleven percent increase between 1978 and 1984.

The declining state of the Beloit Memorial Hospital led the board of trustees to make a leadership change in early 1984. The previous administrator retired and a new president and chief executive officer was recruited. The turnaround that followed my arrival took three years to accomplish. This book is about common sense management approaches which can be applied to any hospital situation regardless of whether a turnaround is necessary. What is most remarkable about our story is that successful results were accomplished with little outside consulting assistance. Common sense approaches in finance, marketing, personnel, and getting close to customers were used. The board, management, physicians and employees all worked hard as an effective team to achieve a real success.

How is success defined? Beloit Memorial Hospital has had its three most financially successful years in its history since the turnaround began. Operating profits in 1984, 1985 and 1986 exceeded $900,000.

Market research studies in 1986 confirm that the hospital's image has significantly improved. Most importantly, the hospital's inpatient and outpatient business is growing again. In 1986, Beloit Memorial Hospital became one of the few hospitals in Wisconsin and around the country whose inpatient census increased. Outpatient business increased at roughly triple the national average.

In the course of our turnaround, mistakes were made. Many are identified for readers to help them avoid reinventing our errors. Each chapter ends with a "hindsight" section which identifies what could have been done differently. Faced with uncertainty, declining business and an overall poor financial situation, success was far from guaranteed. Errors notwithstanding, Beloit Memorial Hospital did succeed.

This book is organized in four sections, covering three years. Our hospital turnaround was not unlike the course of treating a trauma patient. Crisis management came first in year one, much as emergency physicians would approach a trauma patient to achieve stabilization of vital signs. After initiating crisis management strategies, diagnosis of the hospital's problems followed, just as a physician thoroughly evaluates a trauma patient after immediate life threatening problems have been stabilized. Diagnosis gave way to treatment in year two. Finally, year three involved rehabilitation and recovery, much like the trauma patient who survives the initial crisis and treatment. Our patient is recuperating nicely and is stronger for the turnaround ordeal.

No hospital is beyond salvage. Hard work and common sense leadership approaches discussed throughout this book will produce dramatic improvements. If we can do it, any hospital can.

PART I

YEAR ONE: CRISIS MANAGEMENT

Memorable Moment #1:
"I drank Maalox for breakfast—a
whole bottle of it—which I can still
taste three years later when I watch
'60 Minutes' on TV."

CHAPTER ONE

Success Starts with the Board

A HOSPITAL TURNAROUND is not a committee effort. It takes a strong leader to turn around any difficult situation. The board of a troubled hospital should see its role as hiring and retaining the turnaround leader and supporting him when turnaround efforts get into full swing. Beloit Memorial Hospital's Board of Trustees understood this basic fact. They retained the turnaround leader, guided his efforts and let him do his job, setting the stage for success.

It takes an insightful and courageous board to back off and let the turnaround leader do his job. The commitment to do just that is paramount if a turnaround is to succeed. What exactly should the board be prepared for in a hospital turnaround? In two words: major change. It is self-evident that a hospital in need of a turnaround is experiencing major problems. Change will be needed to resolve those problems. The board will be faced with overseeing and supporting changes in virtually every aspect of the hospital's operation. The change process usually begins with selecting new hospital leadership. In Beloit, the board got its first taste of community reactions to come when some of the second guessers focused on the age of the new hospital CEO.

I remember standing in line at the grocery store shortly after arriving in Beloit listening to a ten-minute diatribe by two couples in front of me blasting the hospital board for selecting a virtual teenager to run the local hospital. I was 32 when I arrived in Beloit, a fact the local paper pointed out no fewer than 10 times in various articles during my first week on the job.

SELECTING A NEW LEADER

Beloit Memorial Hospital's Board knew it had to make a leadership change by mid-1983. The accelerating decline of the hospital, worsening financial condition, and the growing unhappiness of the medical staff and employees all confirmed that a leadership change was necessary.

Like many boards, Beloit's used an outside management consultant to confirm the obvious. Report in hand, the trustees retired the previous administrator and initiated recruitment for a new CEO. Their approach was to organize a board search committee. An executive search firm was not engaged. Prospective candidates were generated through word of mouth referrals. I heard of the position from a Wisconsin CEO colleague from a nearby hospital.

My first interview was very interesting. The search committee must not have read the "Personal" section of my résumé, because they were obviously taken aback by my youth. With an arrogance born of not needing a job, I responded that age must not be a guarantee of success since their administrator with two decades of service had not kept the hospital out of trouble. I returned to New York thinking I would never hear from Beloit again. Wrong.

Two months later I was invited for a second visit. This time the search committee was concerned that I was making too much money. I replied that you get what you pay for. I didn't have the guts at the time to repeat one of John Witt's famous lines about executive recruiting: "If you pay peanuts, don't complain if only monkeys apply." Again I returned to New York thinking I would be written off as a brash young overpaid executive who would not fit in with the conservative board of Beloit Memorial Hospital.

Wrong again. Soon thereafter I was invited back for a third and final interview and subsequently offered the job. I later learned that the board had interviewed over 10 "final" candidates, all older and less well paid than I. The other candidates had not been nearly as blunt about specifying that the board would need to reorganize its bylaws to set up an "office of the president" with the powers normally accorded that position in a corporation. There was lively debate during the four-month period from my first interview to the eventual offer. Not only did the debate center on my age and salary, but more importantly my expectations that the board would have to revert to a policy–making board rather than a hands on board intimately involved in operating details, as they had been in the past.

The decision was ultimately made to give the young, well paid and demanding candidate a shot at the job. They were helped along in that decision by a challenge from me. In my last interview, I told the search committee that I wanted total control of the day-to-day operations and for that I would accept total personal risk. I said bluntly, "If you hire me, I'm going to run the hospital. If I don't do it to your satisfaction, fire me, but don't try to tell me how to run it." My bluntness appealed to the board, most of them anyway. So they hired the youngest, highest paid and most demanding of the candidates. I'm still in Beloit, so at least a majority of the board looks back on their selection with satisfaction.

WHAT COMES NEXT?

In order to turn around a troubled hospital successfully, the board and CEO must agree about the power and responsibilities of the CEO from the beginning. This is best done through changes in the hospital's bylaws to ensure that the necessary responsibilities for completing the turnaround are indeed delegated to the CEO. A suggested position description to accomplish this is included in Appendix A. This position description was adopted by Beloit Memorial Hospital's board upon my arrival. It established a complete change in operating attitude by the board and acknowledged that the previous "administrator/caretaker" system had not produced a healthy organization.

In addition to bylaw changes, the board should make a front end commitment to the CEO that he is going to lead the hospital. This may mean some fundamental changes in the way the board has operated in the past. Sometimes, as hospitals deteriorate, board members respond by trying to get in and help run day-to-day operations. This inevitably makes the situation worse. This happened in Beloit, just as it has in hundreds of troubled hospitals around the country. It didn't work.

If the board is satisfied with the turnaround leader's performance, it should be sure that the CEO is compensated accordingly and has the appropriate fringe benefits commensurate with the risk and responsibilities of the job. My board understood the importance of retention and generously rewarded success. That was to be especially important later because I began getting very generous offers from other hospitals in trouble within a year of my arrival in Beloit, when word of our early turnaround measures began getting around the Midwest. When the turnaround CEO is in place, the board should also be prepared for strongly supporting its change agent. This is no small task. Beloit Memorial Hospital's Board experienced many difficulties in the transition. What follows is a sample of those changes it faced and how it responded.

MANAGEMENT CHANGES

It is usually a foregone conclusion that the CEO will change in a turnaround. Beyond that, the board should be prepared for major changes in management throughout the hospital. It is likely that some or all of the top management will either abandon the hospital because of its difficult situation or be replaced by the new CEO. Further, it is likely that department directors and supervisory positions will experience high turnover. It is also to be expected that a new leader may want to implement organization changes to tailor the organization to his or her leadership style.

The board of a troubled hospital should expect significant changes in staffing levels of their hospital. It is likely that layoffs will be necessary in order to regain financial stability, and that the job descriptions and expectations may be substantially changed for employees. In our turnaround, major staff reductions were necessary. These actions precipitated much employee anger and unfavorable media coverage.

At Beloit Memorial Hospital, there were major changes at all levels in management during our three-year turnaround. Initially one third of the management staff was laid off. Then half of those remaining were replaced. The organization design was substantially changed from a pyramidal structure with five layers to a very flat organization, with only two layers between the CEO and hourly staff members.

Changes in the management staff and organization configuration attracted a great deal of negative community attention. In those difficult days, board members were contacted directly by disgruntled members of the community, separated employees and the media. They were prepared, as with the management changes, to refer those inquiries back to the chief executive officer. There was no second guessing of management nor intervention on behalf of special interest groups. This public show of leadership support made it possible for me to give consistent answers to all parties. It also confirmed the board's role as a policy-setting body rather than an arbitrator of employee disputes or defacto media representative.

PHYSICIAN CHANGES

It is rarely the case that a deteriorating hospital situation is caused exclusively by management problems. Problems are usually precipitated by a combination of community, physician and internal problems. To succeed, the CEO must be the clear leader and communicator with all groups, especially the medical staff. Additionally, the board should be prepared for the sensitive issue of physician recruitment, discipline and even the replacement of some existing physicians who are not meeting the quality standards set forth by the hospital. These are serious issues which generate tremendous heat from the medical staff.

The board must be prepared to back whatever recruitment and physician replacement decisions are agreed upon in the board room. The board should participate in those decisions, but once they are made the CEO must be the spokesman. In our turnaround the board made the clear decision that the CEO represented the board to the medical staff. Nevertheless, physicians who were upset with decisions still attempted to get at the CEO through golf course and cocktail party backstabbing. Board members were frequently cornered by angry physicians, especially in the later phases of the turnaround when considerable pressure was being put on physicians to improve local image and physician attitudes.

A typical approach went something like this. An angry internist approaches a trustee at a cocktail party and said, "That Rindler is a complete dictator. He acts like Hitler and wants to control the world and doctors too." When challenged for specifics by the trustee, the usual response was, "Well, he is doing a good job running the hospital, but I just don't like his style." Fortunately for me and for our hospital, this type of behind-the-scenes maneuvering was ineffective because board members always referred the disgruntled physicians to me. A strong and supportive chairman made a tremendous difference in our board's handling of these sticky physician problems.

VENDOR AND SUPPLIER CHANGES

Hospitals in financial trouble must make aggressive efforts to obtain the best possible prices for goods and services to reduce operating expenses. This means that aggressive competitive bidding and major changes in the vendors used for supplies and services may be forthcoming. If this is the case, the board should be prepared for approaches by representatives of those vendors, especially if local vendors are going to lose hospital business. The board should be prepared to refer those comments to the chief executive officer for follow up and not get involved in the operating details of bidding and purchasing decisions of the hospital. To do so compromises the CEO's ability to negotiate the best possible prices. It also leaves board members open for charges of conflict of interest.

The board's role is holding the chief executive officer accountable for obtaining the highest quality goods and services at the best possible prices. It should assess the status of that expectation through its review of financial statements. It should not involve itself in purchasing decisions. If the board has so little confidence in the chief executive officer that it feels it must involve itself in purchasing decisions, then it is obvious that it does not have enough confidence in the leader to execute a turnaround.

During Beloit's turnaround, several local vendors approached individual board members to gain special considerations when they feared losing hospital business. Mostly these special considerations were in the form of getting the hospital to change its mind about purchasing elsewhere because it had found either better prices, better quality or both. Other than passing these comments to me, Beloit's board never tried to influence purchasing decisions. Local vendors quickly got the idea that they must compete for hospital business, not expect to get it as a result of having their next door neighbor on the hospital board.

WHAT SHOULD A TURNAROUND CEO LOOK FOR?

If you are an executive contemplating taking a hospital turnaround assignment, carefully evaluate certain things before accepting the challenge. A thorough evaluation of the hospital board is extremely important. A prospective candidate should start by reviewing the board meeting and committee meeting minutes for at least two years. If board minutes contain lengthy diatribes by board members about their neighbor's complaints about hospital care, or lengthy debates about which insurance company to give the liability coverage business to, that is a signal that the board is more interested in operating details than in being a policy group. Another tip off is the number of committees utilized by the board. If the board utilizes hands on committees like personnel and building and grounds, they want to participate in decisions that are more appropriately handled by the CEO. If the color of the new lobby carpet is the subject of boardroom debate, the prospective CEO should look elsewhere.

Another item to look for is the turnover rate among board members. Is the board made up of individuals who have served for 15 - 20 years? If so, they may think they own the hospital, and this attitude may make it very difficult for a change agent to succeed, no matter how badly change is needed. Also, it is important to review personal ties of board members to businesses and services related to the hospital. Are management ranks populated with board member relatives? Are board members providing goods and services to the hospital through their personal businesses? Are members of the Auxiliary related to board members and physicians? An affirmative answer to any of these questions should require further probing by the prospective CEO to determine whether or not undue influence is being exercised over the operation of the hospital.

Lastly, the prospective CEO should evaluate the leadership strength of the board. A strong board is vital to a successful turnaround. Note that strong does not necessarily mean someone who is adamant about rehiring a next door neighbor who was fired or selecting the color of the wallpaper for patient rooms. Strong in this context means the ability to deflect community questions to the CEO, the ability to provide quality consultation advice to the CEO and the ability to separate details from policy.

It has always been lonely at the top. In a turnaround, it is even lonelier. Personnel and organization tensions run at a peak for months. Sometimes it seems that they are unbearable. It is important to have a board chairman, and perhaps one or two other board members, readily available to the CEO. I was fortunate to have several such board members and an extremely supportive chairman. Their perspective and wise counsel during the dark moments were invaluable.

LESSONS OF HINDSIGHT

The best decision the Beloit Memorial Hospital Board made to ensure the success of its turnaround was to change from the administrator approach, with a high degree of board involvement in day-to-day operations, to the chief executive officer approach. This change of attitude centralized the leadership for our hospital.

A board faced with a turnaround must carefully examine itself. At Beloit, our board did this with the help of an outside consultant. That firm's report helped convince the board that it needed a strong leader to survive. In a different situation, perhaps a hospital already has a strong leader but a weak board which allows physicians, employees or special interest groups like vendors to dictate policy. In that case, it would be the board rather than the CEO that should be replaced. The point is that each hospital situation is different. The board itself must objectively decide where the problems lie and then be strong enough to take whatever action is necessary to resolve these problems.

The hindsight lesson was a personal one. I accepted the CEO position without a significant severance agreement. Knowing what I know now, I would never do that again. A turnaround situation is probably the most risky job a hospital CEO can undertake. A California CEO acquaintance learned that lesson the hard way. In the early 1980s he turned around a financially troubled community hospital in a mere two years. When the hospital was back in the black he was fired because the physicians did not like his heavy-handed management style. The board was not strong enough to put the medical staff in its place and sacrificed an excellent leader rather than confront the medical staff. A separation agreement which provides for at least one or ideally two year's salary in the event of termination should be a prerequisite of any CEO accepting a turnaround assignment. As the American Express commercials say, "Don't leave home without it."

CHAPTER TWO

Downsizing Management

WITH BOARD SUPPORT firmly established, the turnaround began.

Where does a CEO start? Faced with multiple problems, any one of which could be threatening to the continued survival of the organization, it is not so easy deciding where to start. You cannot turn around a hospital without good leadership. Leadership obviously begins with the CEO and top management. The success of Beloit Memorial Hospital's turnaround began with reorganizing and downsizing management.

Immediate management downsizing made an important symbolic statement to the rest of our organization. Changes at the top can lay good groundwork for changes which inevitably are going to be needed throughout lower levels of the organization. Another good reason to start with management downsizing is that the new leadership is going to need the ability to change and communicate quickly. A trimmed down organization is essential to communicate and act fast.

There are two major issues which need to be dealt with regarding management. The first is the organization's design. Reducing the number of organization layers and consolidating positions can and should be done quickly. The approach utilized by Beloit Memorial Hospital is the subject of this chapter. The second issue is evaluating the competence of the individuals who occupy the management positions once the organization design has been settled. Who should be fired? Who should be retained? These questions are discussed in chapter 8.

It was obvious from my first day on the job that Beloit Memorial Hospital had allowed its middle management and its bureaucratic structure to get far too large. Downsizing management became an immediate priority. Reducing salary expenses and sending a signal to the hourly staff that the burden of expense reductions would not fall entirely on them was very important to me. Management was going to share in whatever expense reductions would inevitably take place. I wanted employees to know that and see the proof.

ORGANIZATION DIAGNOSIS: OBESITY

Many hospitals have tended toward organizational obesity in recent years. Beloit was a great example. In their eagerness to act like big business organizations, some hospitals have built up a bureaucracy with many, many layers between the CEO and hourly employees. In a turnaround, a fast and responsive organization is critical. In my judgment, there need not be any more than two layers of management between the chief executive officer and hourly employees in hospitals with 300 or fewer beds. Chief operating officers and staff vice presidents of planning and marketing are a waste of money in a well-led hospital. I believe they exist because too many CEOs see themselves as outside statesmen rather than the individual responsible for running their hospitals. For larger hospitals, no more than three layers are necessary. Further, operating divisions of the hospital should be organized along functional lines rather than around individual likes, dislikes and capabilities.

My approach to evaluating the organizational structure of Beloit Memorial Hospital was to apply common sense and show irreverence for the status quo. Beloit Memorial

Hospital had four vice presidents, an appropriate number for its size. However, the assignment of departments to those vice presidents was eclectic, to say the least. The finance vice president was in charge of departments like central service supply, about which he knew very little. The personnel vice president supervised the physical therapy and respiratory therapy services, about which he knew nothing. The planning vice president supervised a mixture of diverse departments like engineering, laboratory, radiology and food service.

I concluded that four divisions were appropriate; however, the assignment of department responsibilities in the divisions was far from rational. When I asked a senior member of the management how the divisions had been set up, the response was that departments were assigned based on who could get along with whom. Now *there* is a scientific approach if I ever heard one!

After deciding to reassign departments along functional lines, I next analyzed middle management positions. There were too many department heads and supervisors, especially in some of the smaller service areas like community relations and volunteers. These departments did not need full-time directors. I knew that some positions could be eliminated with no compromising of management effectiveness.

More opportunities to downsize the management staff at Beloit Memorial Hospital were discovered in the supervisory ranks. Many departments had been afforded the luxury of assistant department heads and shift supervisors, who were totally unnecessary. For example, the laboratory had a night shift supervisor who supervised only one other individual. I found out how busy he was one night when I made a surprise visit to the lab at 2 a.m. and discovered him studying for his MBA. I soon discovered that he spent far more time studying than doing anything constructive for the laboratory. In fact he usually did this studying out of earshot of the telephone so he would not be disturbed by requests for STAT tests. He consequently was given the opportunity to study in another hospital. The respiratory therapy department had an evening shift supervisor who supervised only two other people.

However, the biggest build-up of middle management bureaucracy was in the nursing department. The nursing department was a five-layer pyramid. Its organization chart is illustrated in figure 2. Imagine a hospital with approximately 100 inpatients having a nursing department with five separate organization layers. This had not happened overnight. It had evolved over a 10-year period and had gone beyond all semblance of reason and common sense. Nursing management was tripping all over itself looking for something constructive to do. Judging from patient and staff perceptions it wasn't succeeding. Patients frequently complained that if we had fewer bosses maybe they could get bedpans and pain medications sooner. Staff nurses were so confused by the organization labyrinth that most of them did not know who they reported to.

A NEW ORGANIZATION

The first step in our organization renewal process was to redefine the operating divisions of the four vice presidents: professional services; finance; nursing; and support services. Departments were reassigned logically to fit into one of these four divisions. Although these moves did not eliminate any administrative positions, it did begin to bring some order to the administrative organization. The resulting administrative organization chart is illustrated in figure 3.

Next I downsized middle management. In the department head ranks, two positions were eliminated completely and their duties reassigned to other individuals. The biggest savings was in the area of reducing supervisory positions. The nursing organization was reconfigured from a five- to a two-layer organization. This made it possible to eliminate the associate director, two assistant directors and four nursing supervisors. It also enabled us to elevate the head nurses to the status of department directors, making them equal in

---
FIGURE 2

Beloit Memorial Hospital
Department of Nursing

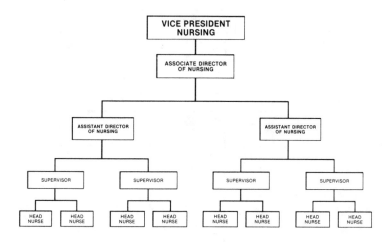

FIGURE 3

Beloit Memorial Hospital
Table of Organization

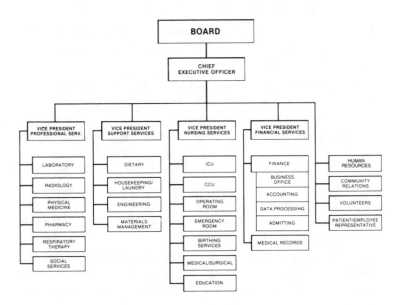

all respects to other department directors throughout the hospital. Additionally, assistant department directors in the radiology department and shift supervisors in the laboratory, respiratory therapy and emergency medicine departments were eliminated. In total, one-third of the management staff positions were eliminated, saving approximately $350,000 in salary expenses.

TEARS, INDIGNATION AND PERSEVERANCE

The decision to eliminate the twelve positions from the management payroll was made by myself and myself only. The vice presidents and department directors had encouraged the build-up of the management bureaucracy. They were ill-equipped to recommend how to dismantle it.

It was not that difficult to select which positions could be eliminated with little or no adverse organizational impact. What was very difficult, however, was deciding what to do with the 12 individuals whose jobs were being eliminated. After much consideration of the obvious options— demotion, transfer or layoff—I elected to lay off all 12. This was a difficult but necessary decision.

It would have been nice to have had the opportunity to get to know the strengths and weaknesses of the 12 individuals whose jobs were being eliminated. It simply was not possible in our turnaround situation because of our precarious finances. The individuals occupying those 12 positions represented a wide range of age, experience, attitudes and competence. There was not time to decide who were the best and who the weakest managers. It was more important to get their salaries off the payroll.

I made the decision to lay off the affected managers without exception. Since the laid off individuals were of all ages and tenure, it was easy to prove that we did not discriminate. This approach enabled us to prevail when the wrongful discharge, race and age discrimination actions were subsequently brought against the hospital. Each of the laid off managers received two weeks' notice and a generous severance pay arrangement. The uniformity of the lay-offs was the single greatest point which enabled the hospital to prevail on all legal actions brought against the hospital. It was a painful decision to separate those individuals. I hope never to be in a position to have to make a decision like that again.

Laying off 12 managers got around town fast. I found out the hard way one afternoon how fast. I was purchasing some running shoes at a local sporting goods store and discovered at the checkout counter I did not have enough cash. When I tried to write a check, the clerk was wary of cashing it because I still had a New York driver's license. He asked me where I worked, and I replied at Beloit Memorial Hospital. For the next 10 minutes he described in detail how that new "son of a bitch president" was firing all the good people and how he was ruining the hospital. When he ran out of breath, he asked me what I did at the hospital. I calmly replied that I was the new son of a bitch president.

LESSONS OF HINDSIGHT

Time has proven the downsizing of our nursing department management staff to be one of our best early changes. It has provided greater upward and downward communication within nursing and enabled us to assign greater accountability and responsibility to head nurses. In any troubled hospital, I venture to guess that a bloated management group is at least partially to blame. While nursing represented the largest target for management reductions in Beloit, a hospital can evaluate its top-heavy position in many other ways. The overdependence on staff positions such as planners, marketers, information system managers and so on is one trap many hospitals fall into. Another is creation of off-shift supervisory positions to oversee only one or two people. A CEO willing to dismantle a status quo organization almost always will be rewarded with substantial salary savings plus a leaner, more efficient staff.

Without question, the decision that could have been made differently was that of not using an outplacement firm. The 12 laid off managers would have benefited from professional counseling. The laying off of those individuals was necessary for the organization's survival. However, outplacement counseling could have eased their transition into new positions and reduced the bad feelings inevitably produced by letting them go.

CHAPTER THREE

Downsizing Staff

$M_{ANAGEMENT}$ downsizing behind us, the next focus was on reducing the employee work force to coincide with patient activity. Staff reductions are painful and disruptive for any organization. In the past several years tens of thousands of employees have been laid off from hospitals throughout the country. If it becomes necessary at your hospital, be prepared for a challenging leadership problem.

In our hospital, staff reductions obviously had to be made. Inpatient census had dropped by 41 percent in five years with practically no changes in the staffing patterns. Employees knew in their hearts that reductions had to be made. Nevertheless, they found it difficult to face reality. The uncertainty created by not knowing when or if a layoff was coming created an interesting morale phenomenon. In talking with CEO colleagues, I am told that our situation was not unique. As census levels declined and staffing levels remained constant, employees' perception of work load increased dramatically. As there was less work to do, Beloit employees felt they were more and more overworked.

Perhaps this was a defense mechanism against inevitable layoffs. A cynic might suggest that there was simply more time on employees' hands to gripe, perhaps that extra time was being spent complaining about their high work load, whereas before that time was used productively. I do not profess to understand the psychology. But it was evident that our employees felt more overworked with less actual work to do.

The first strategy to deal with this hysteria and to lay groundwork for inevitable staff reductions was to communicate. Employees, management and physicians must clearly know the actual status of the hospital. This means communicating verbally and publishing the key activity trends and financial trends for the hospital. There is nothing like honesty and forthrightness for laying the appropriate groundwork for the difficult decisions which surround employee staff reductions. I told management, physicians and employees exactly how much business the hospital had lost, exactly what the financial losses had been, and what could be expected in the future if adjustments were not made. It was a grim message. Either we cut expenses or we go bankrupt. Communicating does not necessarily bring everyone into agreement about how much and what kind of reductions are necessary. But it does establish that changes are needed if the organization is going to survive.

THE FIRST DECISION: HOW MUCH TO CUT?

In a turnaround, overall corporate financial objectives should dictate how much staff cutting is necessary. In Beloit it was simple to determine how much had to be cut. The overall corporate strategy was to break even rather than to continue losing money. I had previously determined that approximately $750,000 in operating expenses could be eliminated through supply, service and management reductions. Our total expense reduction needs in year one were approximately $1.3 million. Therefore, staffing levels had to be reduced by approximately $650,000.

Some turnaround strategists suggest that instead of starting with an overall requirement for dollar cuts, you should instead set up management committees to determine how much can objectively be cut. Rule 58 from Dr. Richard Thompson's book on "Theory I" management expresses my thoughts perfectly on committees.

Theory I cake-baking procedure:

Step 1: Appoint the Cake Committee.

Step 2: Hire the Cake Coordinator to staff the Cake Committee.

Step 3: Develop a written plan. Don't call it "recipe." Name it "Long-Range Plan for Development and Implementation of Cake-Baking Objectives."

Step 4: Establish a confidentiality policy for the Cake Committee.

Step 5: Hire an attorney to review the confidentiality policy.

Step 6: Establish a system of agendas, meetings, minutes and progress reports for the Cake Committee.

Step 7: Stay away from the kitchen!

The judgment of how much staff can be cut is tremendously flexible. I advocate having the CEO determine the overall required staff reductions first, and then asking vice presidents and department directors for advice on when and where to implement them.

Timing of the staff reductions is also important. It does no good to plan a staff reduction strategy for nine months, and then only benefit from it for the remaining three months of the year. Our approach was to plan the staff reduction in sixty days. It was then implemented immediately. This sort of "fast tracking" may lead to a less than elegantly implemented staff reduction, but it gets results quickly. In a turnaround, speed is much more important than elegance.

A review of union contract staff reduction provisions needs to be done at the outset too. Our hospital had a union and the layoff provisions were complicated. Consultation with the hospital's labor counsel was vital to ensure that staffing reduction strategies were implemented in accordance with the applicable union contract provisions.

THE SECOND DECISION: WHERE TO CUT?

There are as many different staffing reduction methodologies as there are CEOs and vice presidents of human resources. The simplest approach is to make across-the-board percentage reductions for each department. In my opinion, this is a gutless approach since different departments and shifts within departments have different activity patterns. Even in a failing hospital, a few departments may be holding their own or even growing. To make an across-the-board cut penalizes those departments unfairly.

A detailed department by department analysis was used to determine where to reduce staff in our hospital. Activity trends and paid hour trends were reviewed for the preceding 24 months for every department. Each department has a measurable activity. In the nursing department, it is patient days. In the physical therapy department, it is treatments. In the laboratory department, it is test procedures. Activity trends and paid hour trends were compared to identify significant disparities. For example, our laboratory paid hours per procedure were growing substantially, while laboratory work load was declining. Paid hours were increasing, but procedures were declining. It was this sort of managerial mentality which contributed to the hospital getting in financial trouble in the first place.

Additionally, American Hospital Association Monitrend studies for each department were utilized to make productivity comparisons with other hospitals. Although Monitrend studies were not used as a definitive decision-making tool, they were useful in identifying departments whose productivity levels were less expensive than those of similarly-sized hospitals in the Monitrend comparison groups. These comparisons helped identify our laboratory, central service department and medical/surgical nursing units as being more overstaffed than, for example, our radiology department, physical medicine department, or pharmacy department.

Meanwhile, special circumstances in each department were reviewed. Some departments are more activity sensitive than others. For example, engineering is less sensitive to swings in the inpatient census than nursing. Dietary, on the other hand, is almost totally influenced by the inpatient census. If there are fewer patients, fewer meals are fixed, requiring fewer staff hours.

Some alarming staffing trends came to light because of these reviews. For example, the professional mix in the nursing department was analyzed and determined to be extremely low, only 25 percent. This information influenced the nursing staff reduction decisions significantly. When the nursing staff was reduced, the decision was made to reduce unit clerks and nurse aides rather than RNs, since the RN mix was already far too low. This was a rather unusual but effective strategy to increase the RN ratio to 50 percent, which was the end result.

THE RICH GROUNDSMAN

Next a detailed, position by position review was conducted in each department. Common sense examples of overstaffing or inappropriate staffing were sought. Several dramatic examples were discovered. Our engineering department had a $34,000 a year "structural engineer" who was actually mowing grass. Upon investigation, I learned that the structural engineer had been hired by the building and grounds committee of the board four years previously to deal with a roofing problem. It took approximately six months for the individual to finish working on the roofing problem for which he was hired. Instead of being laid off, he was retained. He was cutting grass in the summer and shoveling snow in the winter. Don't laugh. More than one board that thought it was doing the right thing has made decisions equally bad.

I also discovered that we had a $35,000 a year Ph.D.

chemist in our laboratory contributing little if anything to the effective operation of the department. To add insult to injury, the gentleman was a farmer who molded his work schedule around his farm schedule. His hours and accountability were extremely erratic. When reviewing a detailed listing of positions, assume nothing and question everything. If you do you might even discover a $34,000 a year sidewalk shoveler or gentleman farmer scientist.

When the department and the individual position analyses were completed, I made the final decisions about how much each department should be cut, or if they should be cut at all. In almost every case, I decided to cut more than the department directors and vice presidents recommended. If I had followed their recommendations exclusively, only $200,000 in staff expense would have been cut, not the needed $650,000. Thirteen departments received staff reductions of varying degrees. Three departments received no staff reductions since it was determined that their activity levels had not declined during the past 24 months and their productivity levels were within reasonable limits. Three departments actually got staffing increases. Their recent growth had been ignored because of the hospital's poor overall financial condition.

When reduction decisions are ultimately made, dollar savings projections must be carefully analyzed to determine if the overall expense reduction goals are being met. This projection is not a simple calculation. It obviously involves projecting the amount of payroll that is reduced. Beyond that it also involves taking into account the unemployment compensation impact and the impact of continuing benefits for varying periods of time which are sometimes necessitated by union contracts or state employment laws.

After our expense reduction decisions were made, it was determined that we would save $650,000 a year as projected. However, for the first six months following the reductions, only about 60 percent of the benefit of the reductions materialized, due to unemployment compensation expenses which partially offset the savings.

REDUCTION STRATEGY QUESTIONS

Just as there are seven questions that the American Cancer Society publishes to enable the public to test themselves for cancer symptoms, there are seven questions the turnaround leader must ask to determine if a layoff is planned effectively.

1. *Do we use layoffs or hour reductions?*
   Our experience suggests that layoffs are better when there is a permanent expectation of a business downturn and no hope of recovery within 24 months. Hour reductions can be used on a temporary basis, but tend to be demoralizing and create attitude problems among the employees whose hours are reduced. A combination of layoffs and hour reductions was used in Beloit. In order to remove 60 full-time equivalents (FTE) from our payroll, 30 full-time people were laid off and the hours of 90 more employees reduced to obtain the remaining thirty FTE reduction.

2. *Should we reduce salaries instead of layoffs?*
   The use of salary reductions is a short term strategy. Employees will accept a short term loss of salary without too much grumbling. Indeed, some of the professional service departments accept salary cuts much better than hours reduction or layoffs, since this gives them the opportunity to continue treating patients in the fashion they have been doing previous to the reduction. However, if the salary reduction goes on too long, for instance for over three months, it may cause the loss of employees who can go elsewhere to work for their original or even higher salaries.

3. *Should you use seniority or competence in layoff decisions?*
   It would be nice to be able to utilize competence in the decision about whom to lay off. However, in our situation the personnel evaluations were so poorly done that there was no way to really tell which employees were more competent than others. Therefore seniority was used. Also, many union contracts specify the use of se-

niority rather than personnel evaluations, and seniority decisions are easier to defend in court than supervisory evaluations.

4. *What about bumping?*

Bumping is the term used to describe the process specified in some union contracts which enables more senior employees to bump employees out of their jobs when layoffs are made. For example, a more senior person in the housekeeping department may bump a less senior one in the dietary department, instead of being laid off. These provisions are extremely disruptive but must be accommodated if bumping is part of the hospital's union contract.

5. *Is there a best day of the week to announce a layoff?*

Probably not. But there is a worst day of the week. To announce a layoff on a Friday afternoon is not a good idea. It leaves the whole weekend for employees to react without having supervisors around to answer questions and deal with inevitable rumors and hard feelings. I recommend that layoff announcements be made early in the week.

6. *What's the dumbest thing a CEO can do prior to or during a staff reduction?*

The dumbest thing a CEO can do is take delivery on a new company car during a layoff. Rumor has it that the entire management of a midwest hospital took delivery of brand new company cars (Cadillacs) the week a nursing cutback was announced. The person who made that decision is an endangered specie.

7. *What's the smartest thing that can be done during a staff reduction?*

The smartest thing any management can do during a staff reduction is to be visible and communicate. There is no substitute for doing it personally, as we'll discuss next.

DAY OF RECKONING

When all the planning is completed, the time comes for swallowing hard and implementing the staff reduction. Before the reduction takes place, there are four key groups who should receive advance notification. It goes without saying that the board should be briefed prior to the implementation of any staff reductions. They should be prepared to refer all questions about the staff reductions to the CEO for follow up. When the board gets involved in trying to answer questions from the media, next door neighbors, physicians or disgruntled employees, it compromises the ability of the CEO to follow through. When questions are received, they should be immediately referred to the CEO, and the CEO should be diligent enough to follow up on them with accurate and concise responses.

The management staff also needs to be fully briefed on the staff reductions prior to the public announcements. I suggest that this be done in person by the CEO to give all supervisors, department directors and administrative staff members an opportunity to ask any questions prior to the time the actual public announcement is made. Thirdly, physicians should be briefed in advance prior to the actual staff reduction. Physicians play an extremely important role in the reduction implementation and the recovery process which the organization will go through following the staff reduction.

Some of my colleagues found it hard to believe that I announced, in a general medical staff meeting, our staff reduction plans ten days before they were announced to employees. I took the physicians into my confidence and explained in detail what was going to happen and why. I was rewarded by a completely confidential attitude on the part of physicians. No physicians leaked the news before the actual staff reductions took place. Advance notice had a great deal to do with creating a positive physician attitude about the reductions and a supportive role during the post reduction recovery process.

Lastly, when it comes time to communicate the reductions to employees, there is no substitute for the CEO doing it personally. After letting each department manager know how the cuts were going to affect his or her specific department, I met personally with all employees on all shifts to explain the reasons for the overall staff reductions and the mechanics for implementing the reductions. These were probably the most terrible seven days that I experienced during the turnaround. Twenty-four meetings were held. As you can imagine there was a great deal of anger, frustration and tears. However, I believe strongly that the leadership gained the respect of our employees by communicating bad news personally and letting them know who made the decisions and why. I told them I had made the decisions personally. I also told them those decisions were vital to the hospital's survival. I didn't like it any better than they did, but it had to be done.

Employees who lost their jobs received two weeks notice. In addition, employees who were having their hours cut also received two weeks' notice. Some hospitals have chosen to communicate the bad news on a Friday afternoon and give the employees two weeks' severance pay but not have them return to work meanwhile. I did not feel that this approach was consistent with our organization's needs. There is a grieving process which takes place when a staff reduction is implemented. Giving the employees several weeks to say goodbye to their friends is an important part of dealing with this grieving process. It is well worth the temporary decline in morale caused by having the "doomed" employees physically on the premises for two weeks. As for the timing of the announcement, I announced the layoffs during the beginning of the week so that supervisors would be available to answer questions and so that top management could be visible following the reduction announcements.

With reference to external communication, a very conservative approach was taken. A brief written news statement for the TV stations and local newspapers was released. The layoff was big news. On the day following the initial news release six TV station cameramen and reporters showed up to interview employees affected and to obtain a statement from management. I will never forget that morning. I drank Maalox for breakfast—a whole bottle of it—

which I can still taste three years later when I watch "60 Minutes" on TV. I felt as though the hospital were under siege by a bunch of young Mike Wallace aspirants who wanted to ask me the definitive question on camera to make the hospital president look like a total jerk. I was confident they could succeed so I declined to comment on camera. In hindsight, I feel that was one of the best decisions in handling the media. To say as little as possible about a bad situation seemed to quicken the time that it took to blow over. To debate with disgruntled employees or union officials on camera or in the newspaper is an exercise in futility and would have extended the layoff's newsworthiness.

A SPECIAL WORD ABOUT PHYSICIANS

To understand the importance of physicians in a staff reduction, imagine this hypothetical story. You are a surgeon listening to a young nurse tell you about her pink slip informing her that she has just been laid off, effective 3 p.m. today, Friday. With tears in her eyes, she tells you how much she loves her job, especially taking care of *your* patients. You cannot believe what you are hearing. How could that hospital administrator be so callous as to lay off one of *your* best nurses? You reassure the nurse that its just another stupid decision by the administrator and you will do everything in your power to get her job back. Although you know that the hospital's census has declined rapidly in the past year, you had no idea that a layoff was imminent. As your anger and indignation rise, you head for the nearest telephone to start calling your board member friends, thinking a few well-placed words can resolve the matter.

More than one physician has been faced with this situation. It can and should be avoided. Physicians can do a great deal to ease the impact of a staff reduction. They are informal leaders and employees pay a great deal of attention to their response to management. There are several constructive physician approaches which will unquestionably assist the hospital. First, physicians should thoroughly understand the need for the staff reductions and the process used to make the layoff decisions. There is an obligation on the hospital's leadership to be sure that understanding is developed.

We were extremely fortunate during our staff reductions that physicians took an active and positive role in making constructive responses to our patients and community. They were well informed, and used the information to be advocates on the hospital's behalf. I recall a particularly satisfying call from a patient who wanted to tell me that an orthopedic surgeon had just spent 30 minutes with him at his bedside explaining the need for staff reductions and reassuring him that no quality of care declines would follow.

THE AFTERMATH

What happens when a staff reduction is implemented? It precipitates many responses, most of them negative. Employees who are directly affected will be predictably angry and negative. Those who are not directly affected will also be upset by the uncertainty of future staff reductions and the overall upset of their colleagues who will be leaving.

In addition to the immediate anger, employees in departments that are affected less or not at all by the layoffs will probably begin complaining about their work loads. This is especially true in nursing units. When our staff levels were reduced, the remaining nursing staff members began expressing to physicians and patients their concerns about being overworked. It was only through high visibility of the head nurses and administrative staff that we learned about the complaining quickly and dealt with it.

The CEO should also be prepared for a tremendous amount of second guessing which takes place in the immediate aftermath of a staff reduction. Although the hospital's declining census and deteriorating financial position may be well known and even well understood, when a staff reduction takes place it is certain that some people will disagree about the need for it or the way it was done. When our staff reduction was implemented, I could not believe how many employees, managers and even Auxiliary members suddenly became experts on how the staff reduction should have been accomplished. The hospital leader should be prepared for this second guessing and try not to get too defensive about it. He should also be prepared for further events like informational picketing and critical editorials, both of which resulted from our layoffs.

Lastly, in the aftermath of the staff reduction the hospital's leadership should take good notes about how the implementation phase succeeded and failed. It might come in handy if you have to go through it again.

LESSONS OF HINDSIGHT

The most important lesson I learned about staffing reductions was from a sister hospital in Wisconsin. It was too late to do our hospital any good. That hospital hired outplacement counselors for employees who were laid off. They helped the employees organize their resumes and their job searches. Unfortunately, we did not do this with our staff, and I regret that omission to this day. Any leader faced with the terrible prospect of a layoff or staff reduction should consider outplacement counseling to help affected employees locate new employment.

CHAPTER FOUR

Reducing Supply Expenses

HOSPITALS WASTE tremendous amounts of money on supplies. The ability to reduce supply expenses intelligently and quickly can speed financial recovery and return the hospital to profitability. Even if a hospital is not in financial trouble, there are many opportunities to save money and reinvest savings for patient care improvements. At Beloit Memorial Hospital, six figure supply savings were achieved in a very short period of time. No magic, just common sense and hardball negotiating.

The key to expense reductions is flexibility. During turnarounds there is a more flexible attitude about trying alternatives among employees and physicians. This translates into a willingness to try new supplies, services or equipment that might normally meet with much resistance. Another key aspect of reducing supply expenses is the ability to negotiate with vendors. This tests the gastric mucosa of any hospital executive just as much as staff reductions, but is eminently more satisfying.

When developing supply reduction strategies, go for the big dollars. In a panic to reduce expenses, some hospitals focus on "nickel and dime" items. The tremendous energy involved in chasing nickel and dime savings diverts attention from opportunities for really big reductions. During the first year of Beloit Memorial Hospital's turnaround, non-salary expense reductions of $400,000 were achieved. None of these reductions diminished the quality of care. Some changes actually increased the quality of services rendered at our hospital. Here is how we did it.

IT'S LIKE PICKING CHERRIES

Early in the turnaround one of our physicians remarked that there were so many opportunities to save money that it would be like "picking cherries." He proved to be absolutely right. The process began by identifying the high expense items. Instead of concentrating on reducing the number of pencils and pens, a thorough analysis of invoices identified the 20 most expensive supply items. Not necessarily most expensive in terms of individual price, but most expensive in terms of total dollars spent during the year.

A relatively expensive item like a $5,000 lithium pacemaker did not make the list since only a handful were implanted each year. On the other hand, relatively inexpensive items like underpads did make the list since hundreds of thousands of those inexpensive items are used per year. Through the analysis of invoices, the materials management department identified our 20 most expensive items: IV solutions, urological supplies, x-ray film, food and others.

The next step was to identify alternative suppliers and vendors for each high expense item. You might assume that this would be happening on an ongoing basis. It should have been. However, our hospital had been not aggressively pursuing alternative suppliers and vendors over the years. Instead, it had become focused on particular brands or vendors out of physician or departmental preference. Needless to say, this approach was not the most cost effective way to purchase supplies.

After identifying alternatives for each high expense supply, a negotiation strategy was developed. In some cases, strategies were based upon implementing new competitive bidding practices. In others they were dependent on developing product standardization approaches. More on that later. The use of competitive bidding must be aggressive if it's going to produce results. Some hospitals think that sending out three bids for an item like surgeon's gloves is an effective process which will achieve best price. This is certainly not the case if powerful surgeons on the staff let the current glove vendor know that there is no way they will change to Brand X. This happens all too frequently when physicians are permitted to speak to vendors directly to express their personal preferences.

At Beloit Memorial Hospital physicians, not hospital management, were controlling major supply decisions. For the most part, physicians could not have cared less what the hospital paid for a supply, as long as they got their preference. All too frequently purchasing executives did not have administrative support to face off with physicians and separate personal preference and bias from effective decision making.

What follows are a few mini-case studies which give specifics on how supply expenses were reduced at Beloit Memorial Hospital.

1. *X-Ray Film*

   Like many hospitals, the dominant brand x-ray film was used at Beloit Memorial Hospital; radiologists refused to consider alternatives. They claimed that there was a definite quality difference between the dominant brand film and the available alternatives. We decided to put this opinion to a scientific test. For one month, three alternative films were tested. All three brands were placed in unmarked coded boxes. Only the chief technologist knew which brand was which. During the month, radiologists made evaluative comments about the quality of each of the three types of film, not knowing the actual brand names of the film they were using. At the end of the month, it was clear that neither radiologists nor the technicians could tell any quality difference in the three films.

   Following this evaluation, new competitive bids were obtained. It was made clear to our current vendor

that a blind evaluation proved that there was no discern-
able quality difference in any of the three films. This was
a major psychological blow for the vendor. In the end,
the hospital saved approximately $25,000 per year based
on that competitive bid.

2. *Intraocular Lenses*
By competitively bidding the intraocular lens account,
our materials management department saved $20,000
per year. There are strong physician preferences on the
use of intraocular lenses, especially from the eye surgeons, who were kept out of the negotiation process. All
vendors were convinced that there was an equal chance
of getting our business. This caused our existing vendor,
which thought it had the business locked up forever because of physician preference, to drop its price by approximately $20,000.

3. *Disposable Dishes*
Another common sense approach to reduce supply expenses was eliminating disposable items on patient meal
trays. Our hospital had lapsed into the practice of using
disposable plates, disposable knives, forks and spoons,
and disposable drinking cups for its dietary service. In my
judgment, this is a disgrace. Hospital patients are paying a
high price for hospital services. They deserve better quality items to eat their meals with than fast food plasticware.

Years ago, our hospital dietary director had been
convinced by a creative salesman that a great amount of
money could be saved by going to disposables. He quoted
the number of man hours that would be saved each year
and the breakage of glassware that would be reduced.
The fallacy of this reasoning was that when the hospital
switched to disposables it did not reduce man hours to
achieve any actual savings. Instead of laying off the dish-
washers, the dietary department found other duties for
the staff. Therefore, the staff expense stayed the same,
and the hospital actually incurred additional costs because disposable dinnerware is quite expensive. Perhaps
that's the reason why most households do not use dispos-

able dinnerware to eat from every day of the week. If we don't do it in our homes, why should we do it for our patients?

Purchasing real china plates, glassware, thermal pitchers for coffee and stainless steel flatware significantly improved the quality of meal services for our patients. The coffee stayed hotter in thermal reusable containers far longer than it did in the old styrofoam cup and flimsy lid combination. Patients found it easier to eat their meals with real stainless steel knives and forks and plates than with the old plasticware. It was especially easier to cut the tough, low quality meat being served at the time.

Not only was the quality of the dinner service improved, but the appearance of the meal trays improved as well. And the real bonus was the $10,000 a year savings earned by getting the dishwashers back in the dishwashing room without adding any staff expenses. Miraculously, the duties that they were performing elsewhere got done anyway. Everyone in the kitchen pitched in and worked harder.

4. *Urology Supplies*

Our hospital had only one urologist at the beginning of the turnaround. Because of his personal preferences, urology supplies had never been competitively bid to alternate suppliers. By keeping the urologist out of the bidding process and by evaluating alternative systems, the hospital was able to save over $25,000 a year. No change of vendors took place as a result of this competitive bid. The existing vendor dropped its price by $25,000 immediately just because competitive bids were implemented. The vendor knew that the urologist could no longer guarantee the business.

5. *IV Solutions*

IV solutions are a high expense item in any hospital. IV purchases are often part of a group purchasing contract. A valuable lesson was learned by shopping the contract directly to IV manufacturers in addition to evaluating options provided under our group purchasing agreements.

We saved $20,000 per year by dropping our group pur-
chasing arrangement and purchasing our IV solutions directly from the manufacturer. Anyone who thinks that
group purchasing arrangements are a panacea is naive.
They are not.

Why? I had learned the answer in a previous job.
While involved in purchasing IVs through a large group
purchasing organization in New York, I decided to get
separate bids from the manufacturers. I was astounded
that I was able to negotiate a better deal than the purchasing group, which had 3,000 beds in purchasing power behind it. When I pursued the matter I learned that
sometimes manufacturers do not offer the best deals to
groups because of the slow payment pattern of some financially strapped members. By offering prompt payment guarantees to the manufacturer, I was able to beat
the prices of the large group. It left me with the impression that large purchasing groups are only as strong as
their weakest members.

6. *Underpads*
Underpads, disposable absorbent towel-like items, are
high expense items because of the number used on an annual basis. When underpad expenses were evaluated, a
valuable lesson about buying for quality rather than just
price was learned.

In evaluating existing underpads, it was determined
that the low bid had been purchased for years. The low
bid was the flimsiest and lowest quality item among the
alternatives. They were of such low quality that the nursing staff was using two or three underpads each time a
patient required one. Underpad usage had doubled and
tripled over the years. By choosing the lowest quality
item, the purpose of obtaining the best possible value for
underpad products was defeated.

Common sense confirmed that underpad expenses
could be decreased by purchasing one of the most expensive underpads on the market. This underpad was of such
high quality that our nursing staff trusted using only one
at a time. By increasing the quality of a supply item, the
hospital decreased the overall annual cost of underpads

by $10,000. The real lesson was that evaluation of products by the users *after* a decision is made is an important part of intelligent purchasing. Had the original underpad decision been evaluated more carefully it would have been determined that the nurses were using two or three items each time rather than only one, thereby increasing expenses rather than decreasing them.

7. *IV Controls*
Another important strategy for expense reduction proved to be the use of employee supply evaluation teams. A team of nurses evaluating the disposable flow meters on IV lines identified an alternative to our existing product which saved over $25,000 a year. The technical expertise required to make this decision was at the bedside, not in the materials management department. The nursing staff was willing, even eager, to help because they knew savings were being reinvested in improving the quality of equipment and fundamentals. The money saved on IV flow meters was used to purchase electronic thermometers for all nursing units. The new thermometers made life easier on nurses and patients alike.

8. *Medications*
A careful review of our formulary identified several immediate opportunities to reduce drug expenses. This required the assistance and cooperation of physicians. Physicians are threatened when the hospital's viability is uncertain. Our physicians were more willing to be flexible and we took advantage of this cooperative attitude.
Specifically, more generic substitutes were used than had been the hospital's practice previously. This alone saved approximately $50,000 per year. An additional $25,000 was saved by educating physicians about the use of first, second and third generation antibiotics. Our physicians had lapsed into the habit of using the most expensive antibiotic medication rather than some of the inexpensive alternatives which have the same desired results. Through education and generic substitution of antibiotics, the pharmacy was able to significantly reduce antibiotic expenses.

The list goes on and on. Approximately $400,000 was saved in our overall supply budget within a matter of months. Savings were achieved by the use of aggressive competitive bidding, common sense evaluation of alternatives and hardball negotiation strategies. These savings had immediate impact on our bottom line and helped speed our financial turnaround to a successful conclusion.

LESSONS OF HINDSIGHT

The biggest hindsight lesson learned in reducing supply expenses is to assume nothing. Don't assume physicians won't change supplies. Don't assume there is only one best value for the dollar. Don't assume managers and purchasing departments can always spot the best deal. Above all, don't assume that group purchasing arrangements and price vendor contracts achieve the greatest savings for individual hospitals. Our hospital proved time and time again that aggressive purchasing and considering all the options proved to be a far more effective strategy than relying on the easy use of group contract and price vendor arrangements.

CHAPTER FIVE

Reducing Service Expenses

DRAMATIC SERVICE expense reductions were achieved using the same techniques used to reduce supply costs. Identifying the most expensive service contracts came first. Next the alternatives to each of those contracts were investigated and competitive bidding and negotiation strategies followed. A common sense evaluation of various service systems was also undertaken. The result: $250,000 in service expense savings.

For service contracts, like supplies, there had been little aggressive competitive bidding in prior years. Our hospital had fallen into the trap of developing a comfortable relationship with service vendors and did not really keep them on their toes by periodically evaluating options. Inevitably, this led to paying a higher price for services than was necessary.

HOW MUCH IS TOO MUCH?

In addition to evaluating alternatives, a hard look was taken at whether services rendered were producing any useful outcomes for patients. We determined that some purchased services were not producing anything of value for our patients. These were discontinued. A few mini-case studies of successful approaches for reducing service expenses follow:

1. *Accounting Services*
   Like many hospitals, Beloit had developed a comfortable relationship with its audit firm. This relationship had extended for nearly 10 years. During that period there had been no attempt to competitively bid accounting services. A miraculous thing happened when we developed a "Request for Proposal" which had specific performance expectations attached to it and sent it to all the big eight accounting firms. Quotes were returned with prices approximately one third less than we had been paying. This was a clear case of laziness on the part of our organization which led to paying far more for a service than was necessary. Ten thousand dollars were saved by changing audit firms.

2. *Liquid Oxygen Service*
   Liquid oxygen represented an example of where the hospital had been lulled into a false sense of security by staying with a local vendor. The vendor had enjoyed the business for many years. Although the appearance of competitive bids was given, that did not really happen. In fact, several years prior to the turnaround, when the local vendor was about to lose the business because his prices weren't competitive, he went to the purchasing agent and administration and threatened to contact his board friends if he was not allowed to keep the business. Administration caved in to the pressure and the local vendor retained the business, even though his prices were higher. The board never found out. This subsequently discouraged outside vendors from even submitting liquid oxygen quotes to our hospital.
   By rebidding the liquid oxygen service business fairly, the hospital was able to save approximately $10,000 a year. The vendor chosen was located 100 miles away and was still able to serve our account at $10,000 less than a local vendor. I believe in favoring local vendors when all other things are equal. But I could never support paying $10,000 more for a $50,000 annual expense just to keep the business in town.

3. *Rental Services*
   Sometimes hospitals in financial trouble defer capital pur-

chases. This had definitely happened in Beloit. One dramatic example demonstrated the fallacy of deferring needed capital purchases. The hospital had experienced a major increase in demand for IV flow pumps. It had not been able to afford to purchase enough to meet the daily demand. However, since the medical staff continually complained about the shortage of IV flow pumps, the materials management department capitulated by renting IV pumps continuously at a cost far greater than purchasing them in the first place.

Discontinuing the rental of IV pumps and purchasing enough to meet the ongoing need saved $20,000 a year in rental expenses. There were other areas in which the use of short-term rentals were found to be extremely expensive. Purchasing equipment may mean a commitment up front in capital expense but in many instances saves in the long run on operating expenses.

4. *Dues and Network Fees*
This is a touchy subject. The necessity of remaining in state and national associations was evaluated as part of our expense reduction investigations. It was concluded that belonging to the state hospital association was in our continued best interest because of their many valuable services. On the other hand, belonging to national hospital associations and networks did not produce anything of value for our patients in the short run. Although there is nothing inherently wrong with the national networks and associations, during a financial crisis like ours discontinuing memberships and saving the substantial dues is an appropriate cost reduction strategy. Approximately $15,000 per year was saved by dropping several national association memberships.

5. *Maintenance Contracts*
Another area in which substantial savings were achieved was maintenance contracts. Our CT scanner, elevators and HVAC systems all had very expensive maintenance contracts. It was determined that these maintenance contracts had not been competitively bid for some time. By identifying alternative services and by releasing competitive bids, the hospital was able to save approximately

$25,000 per year. Department directors proved to be particularly effective in achieving savings when told that the savings could be reinvested in others areas of their operations to improve quality.

As with supplies, tremendous opportunities exist to save money in the acquisition of services. In some cases, like switching accounting firms, the quality of the service went up at the same time that the price for the service went down. This was possible because Beloit had not been aggressively pursuing its options over the years. I venture to say that nearly all hospitals could benefit from a hard look at their service expenses and a reconsideration of their value in light of alternatives.

MANAGEMENT CONTRACTS: DO IT YOURSELF

In the early days of our turnaround, one major service contract was identified which represented a tremendous opportunity for expense reduction. Like many medium size hospitals around the country, Beloit had lapsed into the practice of using outside management services for some departments. The growth of outside contractors providing housekeeping and laundry management service, pharmacy management services, physical therapy management services and so on had been phenomenal. In some situations, these services can be extremely beneficial. In other situations, they contribute little to the effective and efficient operation of the hospital. Personally, I think the growth of outside firms which manage departments is a function of laziness by hospital executives and a tribute to the marketing skills of the contract companies.

Our hospital was using a prominent service management firm to provide housekeeping and laundry management services, as well as biomedical engineering services. Annual expenses for these three management services exceeded $300,000 per year. The services had been provided by the same firm for 15 years. During that period, we had not investigated competitive bidding or the possibility of providing these services ourselves.

The value of these management services was critically reviewed. I concluded that the service was only worth approximately $200,000. Anything more than that justified us doing it ourselves. With that in mind, I told our contract firm that an immediate price reduction of $100,000 was needed in order for them to retain our contract. You could almost see the tears streaming down their faces. Reference was made to the 15 years of fine service and the high quality of their management team. I responded that those high quality managers seemed to turn over every year or two and that $300,000 was no longer affordable no matter how much we liked the firm or how long they had serviced us.

To make a long story short, the firm conceded and made the $100,000 reduction two weeks later. They were very cooperative and understanding. Their willingness to work with us was appreciated. On the other hand, I could not help wondering how they could reduce the price by $100,000. This negotiation led to the most dramatic one-time savings during our turnaround. It was a hollow victory, however, considering that the hospital might have been overpaying for the last 15 years for a service it could have done internally all along.

Eighteen months later, the management contract firm was separated completely and the hospital saved an additional $50,000 while at the same time improving the overall quality of our housekeeping, laundry and biomedical services.

There may be a place for management contract services in some hospitals. However, I think others have become lazy and have delegated too much of their operation to outside management firms. There are inherent weaknesses in those firms. One is that there tends to be a high turnover of managers, especially in a medium size hospital like ours. Our experience was that the department director for housekeeping and laundry stayed with the hospital for a year or two and then moved up to a bigger hospital as his career developed.

This left very little management continuity in the house-keeping and laundry department. Management contract services are in business to make a profit. That profit is added to the hospital's operating expenses. Medium sized (50-300 beds), competently led hospitals should be able to hire and retain their own directors for all departments rather than depend on outside management contracts to do it for them. The result: lower costs and increased management continuity.

SYSTEM EXPENSES: COMMON SENSE APPLIES

During our turnaround many opportunities were identified to modify and improve systems which improved the quality of services rendered while reducing operating costs. Both large and small systems were evaluated. The savings from common sense changes were impressive.

When Beloit Memorial Hospital was designed during the late 1960s, the automated cart delivery system fad was in full swing. Beloit's architects joined the bandwagon. During my first couple of weeks on the job, I was walking around one Saturday afternoon on the fifth floor, a shelled-in space used for storage and equipment only, when I came upon what appeared to be a dumbwaiter door. As I approached the door it opened all of a sudden and startled me. I let out a not-so-subtle exclamation which startled a nearby employee leaning against a window dozing. When he heard my curse he immediately awoke and came to my assistance. When I asked him what he was doing, he said it was his job to watch the automated carts function during the luncheon meal service. I asked him why. He responded that the system broke down so frequently that it required someone on the fifth floor to monitor it constantly.

A thorough probing of the particulars of our automated dietary delivery system followed. Over the next several days the entire automated loop was traced. The dietary department was located on the third floor of the hospital. Meals were assembled there on a conventional tray assembly line and put into special automated carts. These carts went up to the fifth floor using a dumbwaiter system. On the fifth floor they were sorted "automatically" and then sent to another dumbwaiter on the other side of the floor. The meal trays were then returned to the other side of the third floor of the hospital where the patients are located. This entire process took about 12 minutes. It takes only about 60 seconds to walk food carts from one end of the third floor where dietary is located to the other end where patients are located.

After a thorough 60 second management evaluation, I discontinued the use of the automated tray delivery system and saved $50,000. How? The system broke down so frequently that it required a $25,000 a year maintenance contract which was immediately discontinued. In addition, another $25,000 in man-hour expense was saved by laying off the individuals who dozed on the fifth floor while they were supposed to be watching the carts go by, three meals a day, seven days a week, 52 weeks a year.

The $50,000 savings was then reinvested to improve the quality of the food in the dietary department. This had some immediate positive results for our patients. A hot breakfast was served for the first time, and the quality of the meat was improved. Having real knives and better meat really made our patients happy. The staff was happier too. What a great example of reducing expenses and improving quality at the same time. Not to mention the fact that the new "system" got meals to our patients in a minute or two, rather than twelve or thirteen minutes with the automated system. You can bet that the food was a lot hotter when the old manual system of pushing the carts was used instead of putting them into a magnificent automated system. "Untouched by human hands, untouched by common sense" could have been the design theme for the automated wonder.

There were also some big successes in evaluating small systems. For example, disposable water pitchers were banned from the bedside. These water pitchers, used by many hospitals, are another disgrace. They have several important characteristics. They cost about $1.50 each and they look like plastic junk. They only keep ice water cold for an hour or two. They then begin to sweat all over the bedside stand and produce a small puddle of water suitable for slipping in, causing a patient or staff member to fall. Then, to make matters worse, patients take these flimsy disposable water pitchers home to remind them of how cheap we are.

High quality thermal water pitchers were purchased and substituted for the cheap disposable ones. By doing so, the nursing staff was assisted, since the ice water stayed cold all day long, instead of needing to be changed every hour or two. At the same time the hospital saved about $5,000 a year. Another system savings example is the use of reusable operating room case pans versus disposable wrappers. We saved $10,000 per year in operating costs by buying high quality stainless steel reusable case pans. It required an initial investment of $5,000. We discontinued forever the use of disposable wrappers as an ongoing expense. An additional quality benefit also materialized because the stainless steel case pans have a much longer shelf life than the disposable wrappers.

LESSONS OF HINDSIGHT

Our experience confirmed that there are tremendous opportunities to reduce supply and service expenses while maintaining or even improving service quality. Our energies were not focused on nickel and dime expense items. The big dollar areas were addressed, which required the full cooperation of our employees and medical staff. In a turnaround situation that cooperation is more likely to be there, rather than when things are going great. Take advantage of it while you can.

Another important lesson to remember when cutting costs is never to compromise on quality. Don't fall into the trap of cutting quality with no reference to its impact on patients and staff. Don't purchase toilet paper so cheap that it has wood chips in it unless you want to be accurately labeled an idiot by your patients, employees and physicians. Don't compromise on the quality of food or anything that comes into contact continuously with your customers. If you do, you are asking for trouble. On the other hand, hospitals can intelligently cut costs and actually improve the quality of services and supplies, as our results proved. The creditibility of the turnaround management can be enhanced by reinvesting dollars saved into quality improvements elsewhere in the hospital.

Looking back on our early service expense reductions, one key decision could have been made better. If we had separated ourselves from our housekeeping and laundry management agreement immediately, an additional $50,000 in savings would have materialized. In hindsight, I wish I had gone all the way instead of just negotiating a better price with the service contractor and giving them another year.

PART II

YEAR ONE: DIAGNOSIS

Memorable Moment #2:
"She tearfully described the overwhelming
negative sentiment. She continued by
stating that these were the two worst focus
groups that she had ever conducted during
her 15 year career as an industry and
healthcare market researcher. The next
morning, when I started for work, my first
inclination was to call my former boss in
New York to find out if my old job had
been filled."

CHAPTER SIX

Getting the Outside Picture

IN A HOSPITAL turnaround, the board, management, physicians and employees are very defensive about the decline of their organization. They are not likely to acknowledge that they may have had something to do with the decline. Instead, there is a tendency to point fingers at each other and assign blame. Figure 4 is an illustration of what might have taken place if the board, medical staff, management and employees were all in the same room at the time of my arrival at Beloit Memorial Hospital.

A CEO interested in a turnaround needs to quickly understand finger pointing for what it really is—meaningless. The first constructive step in obtaining an objective assessment of why the hospital got into trouble in the first place is to ask the customers. At Beloit Memorial Hospital, this objective information gathering was accomplished through market research. This approach proved to be one of the most important factors in our ultimate success. It also gave us an objective baseline against which to measure future progress. Here is how we started.

SELECTING A MARKET RESEARCH CONSULTANT

A number of options exist for a hospital to conduct research among their customers. Large hospital consulting firms have

FIGURE 4

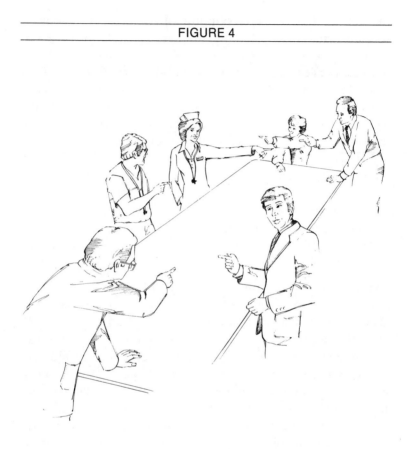

It's Not My Fault!

marketing divisions. Accounting firms have management service arms which handle market research. Advertising firms have market research capability and have lately been increasing their share of the hospital market research business. University marketing professors sometimes provide services on a part-time basis to business and hospital organizations. Lastly, a number of specialized healthcare marketing research and consultation firms are available.

Two capabilities stood foremost in making our decision about which type of consultant to hire. Experience in healthcare market research was a critical factor. The capability within the firm to synthesize the market research information into sound consulting advice was also important. With these two objectives in mind, the option which best met our needs was a healthcare market research firm. The Rynne Marketing Group of Evanston, Illinois, was selected. I look back upon this decision as one of the most important in our turnaround. Rynne Marketing had been in business several years prior to being engaged by our hospital. Their principals were experienced both in industry and healthcare market research, and had hands on hospital management experience which helped them provide high quality consultation advice.

WHAT DID WE NEED TO KNOW?

After engaging our market research firm, we began deciding what we needed to learn most from the research process. We decided that three essential questions had to be answered:

1. How many people were leaving Beloit for hospital services elsewhere?

2. Why were they leaving?

3. For those individuals still utilizing Beloit Memorial Hospital, were they satisfied with our services?

Recall that Beloit Memorial Hospital had lost 41 percent of its inpatient business from 1978 through 1984. The community population increased slightly during that period and unemployment decreased. The only logical explanation was that individuals were leaving the community for hospital care. Some cynics suggested the possibility that the community all of a sudden had become healthy and no longer needed hospital care. But logic prevailed and we looked further.

Beyond the basic questions of out-migration and patient satisfaction, it was important to discover how our community was evaluating the quality (or lack) of hospital services. It was unknown which aspects of care such as room amenities, price, nursing attitude, physician attention, etc., were most important in determining quality perceptions. It was also important to learn how Beloit compared with competing hospitals.

Finally, specific insights into how our current customers perceived key services such as emergency medicine, surgery, maternity, cardiac care, and rehabilitation were included in the study.

MARKET RESEARCH APPROACH

The market research firm developed a two-tiered research approach to obtain the answers to the three critical questions. First, qualitative techniques utilizing focus groups were applied. Two focus groups of Beloit residents were randomly selected and interviewed. The first group was comprised of individuals who had utilized the hospital within the past two years. The second group was comprised of individuals who had used a competing hospital within the past two years. A discussion guide was developed which elicited strengths and weaknesses of our hospital vs. competing hospitals, as well as tested various new program ideas.

I will never forget the evening phone call I received at home from Mary Moosebrugger, who conducted these first focus groups. She tearfully described the overwhelming negative sentiment. She continued by stating that these were the two worst focus groups that she had ever conducted during her 15 year career as an industry and healthcare market researcher. The next morning, when I started for work, my first inclination was to call my former boss in New York to find out if my old job had been filled. It had.

Following the focus groups, a quantitative study was conducted in the community. The objective was to obtain results which would have a confidence interval of plus or minus 5 percent. This necessitated a sample of 350 community residents, using random sample phone survey techniques. The survey questionnaire itself was very comprehensive and the phone interviews took about twenty minutes. It was the first healthcare market research conducted in Beloit. The results of the quantitative research and the focus groups were to play a major role in our turnaround efforts. That is, after we got over the initial shock of the negative findings and were able to think constructively about what to do next.

MOMENT OF TRUTH

My first big moment of truth with the board happened during my third month. As part of my monthly report on operations I casually announced that I had hired a market research firm to conduct a comprehensive community survey. Silence fell over the board room. After a few moments, one trustee asked, "How much is that going to cost?" I responded that the study would cost $35,000. More silence.

During my first several months, my board reports focused on cuts. I was cutting management expenses, laying off excess employees and cutting supply and service expenses. They thought that was great. Now I was spending money on marketing consultants, without their approval. That was a different matter. Prior to my arrival the board was involved in virtually all spending decisions. The previous administration would not have even considered hiring a consultant without board approval. I was just the opposite. I would not have considered asking for board permission for an expense I felt was necessary. A major principle was at stake. I asserted that it was my job to achieve overall final objectives set by the board. The objective in year one was clear—get the operation out of the red. How I achieved the objective was up to me as CEO, in my judgment at least. I felt my responsibility was to report, not request.

There were a few board members clearly opposed to this approach. But, to their credit, they kept their counsel. I knew that my credibility and future were on the line. At the same time, I believed in my judgment and that I could achieve the overall board objective of returning the hospital to profitability. I subsequently did just that and even the most conservative board members began to get used to setting overall financial policy rather than deciding on financial details. That question about marketing consultants was the first and last time I was challenged about spending money.

LESSONS OF HINDSIGHT

Looking back on our first efforts to use market research, the insight is crystal clear. The use of methods like quantitative random sampling carried a scientific credibility among the medical staff that we had not anticipated. The survey results were uniformly negative. However, rather than getting defensive, physicians accepted the results and were much more willing to assist with the necessary changes than they might have been if those recommendations had come solely from management or the board. Market research gave a much needed credibility to our desire to initiate change. For that reason alone it was well worth the expense and effort.

On the down side, physicians could have been more involved in the questionnaire development. This could have been accomplished without compromising the quality of the questionnaire, and might have converted a few of the diehard physicians who thought that market research was a new form of voodoo management.

CHAPTER SEVEN

Getting the Inside Picture

THERE ARE THREE internal groups which can contribute to a hospital's decline: physicians, employees and management. To understand why a hospital is failing, it is vital to obtain an objective assessment of each group's strengths and weaknesses. Beloit Memorial Hospital used a combination of approaches to objectively assess these groups.

As with the outside assessment, there was a tremendous amount of finger pointing with inside groups. Physicians blamed poor management for the hospital's decline. Management blamed the hospital's decline on the poor attitude of physicians and the absence of needed medical specialists. Employees blamed both poor management and poor physician care for the hospital's troubles. The only thing that all three groups agreed on was that the hospital's problems were at least partially caused by high unemployment, low population growth and a depressed economy. None of the three groups had any insight that the hospital's problems could be blamed on their own poor performance and attitude.

An objective assessment does not mean listening to the loudest physician, the most articulate manager or the employee who whines most convincingly. It means systematically gaining input from each of these three groups. Here is how we went about obtaining that input.

UNDERSTANDING PHYSICIAN ISSUES

Several objectives were identified to assess physicians. First, we identified the importance of operational problems which affected physicians. What were the satisfiers and dissatisfiers which needed to be addressed in order to help physicians focus more on quality patient care? Next, we obtained the medical staff's own assessment of its clinical strengths and weaknesses was needed. Third, we learned physicians' reactions to new program suggestions that were being considered was desired.

Two approaches were used to obtain the desired insights. The market research firm conducted focus groups with physicians as a start. Three focus groups were conducted, each attended by approximately 10 physicians. Participation in the focus groups was voluntary and confidential. Two thirds of our medical staff chose to participate. Tempers occasionally flared during the focus groups. However, the insights gained proved invaluable. They identified operational problems, physicians' assessments of the hospital management strengths and weaknesses, and provided an inside assessment of the medical staff's own strong and weak points.

The second approach was stolen from a Chicago hospital also in the midst of a turnaround. Techniques used by George Purvis, executive vice president of Columbus Medical Center in Chicago, were adopted. He had divided key members of his medical staff into small groups and assigned them to his vice presidents. The vice presidents then adopted their assigned physicians and sought them out personally to identify hospital strengths and weaknesses, medical staff strengths and weaknesses, and operating problems associated with their hospital practices. This approach was also used in Beloit. It provided additional insights not brought out by the focus groups. Much of the information gained from these interviews confirmed that the focus group's points were valid and in need of attention.

UNDERSTANDING EMPLOYEE ISSUES

The need for better two-way communication between management and employees was immediately apparent upon my arrival at Beloit Memorial Hospital. During my first days, when meeting informally with small groups, an employee rather emotionally said that she felt there was absolutely no effective communication between management and employees. I asked her for an example and was stunned by her response. She said the hospital had laid off a small number of employees a year previously and employees had learned about the layoff by reading it in the local newspaper. There was no communication with employees beforehand. From that moment on I vowed not to be defensive about employees' perceptions about poor communication. The perception was also fact. I also vowed never to let employees learn about a major news item from the newspaper before they learned it from me.

As with physicians, several objectives for gaining a better understanding of employee issues were formulated. Understanding employees' perception of the hospital's quality of care and patient service was desired. Gaining a better understanding of operational problems as they applied to employees and enlisting their ideas for improvement was also needed. Creating a sense of confidence that employees could have ownership in the hospital's turnaround was considered vital.

Two strategies were initiated to better understand employee issues. I started with a series of management communication initiatives which opened up more two-way communication between top management and employees. Assembly meetings came first. These were quarterly "state of the union" meetings to inform employees about the status of the hospital and upcoming problems and initiatives. Attendance at these meetings was required rather than elective. It has been my experience with meetings of this sort that the employees most needing the communication are the ones least likely to attend elective meetings. On the other hand, required attendance meetings cause some poor attitude employees to complain that they are being taken away from patient care. You can't win.

I decided to require attendance at assembly meetings and err on the side of overcommunication rather than not reach all our staff with important messages. I also decided to pay people to attend these meetings if they could not be scheduled within their normal working day.

Assembly meetings were also structured as two-way communications. I always had a series of messages and information to disseminate. Time at each meeting was reserved for questions, comments, rumors and so on. It takes a while to establish enough mutual trust so that a two-way communication can truly be established. However, with some patience and understanding by the CEO the question and answer period at the end can be as productive, if not more productive, than the formal information dissemination. But a word of caution is necessary. If you open the meeting for questions, you should be prepared to be forthright and answer all questions no matter how difficult or controversial. The question I recall most vividly from my first assembly meeting was, "Are you going to bring your entire management staff from New York with you?" I answered simply, "No." I was tempted to say they would not have wanted anything to do with a hospital which had so many problems.

Many other interesting rumors surfaced during those early assembly meetings. I was asked if a nurse had really been fired for taking home a medication cabinet key. I responded no, she had been fired for stealing medication. Another employee asked if I was going to lay off everyone over age 30. I responded no, because I would have had to lay off myself. Another memorable rumor was that all nurses were going to have to wear caps again. I said that I was a brave hospital president, but not brave enough to require caps.

One employee even asked me if my car (a red Porsche 911) had been paid for with hospital funds. After I stopped laughing, I reassured the employee that the Porsche had been paid for while I worked in New York.

In addition to the assembly meetings, I also implemented a "president's exchange." This was a monthly forum which permitted me to address small groups of employees and give them a detailed briefing of the hospital's status. These briefings contained the same information that was disseminated to the medical staff and board. It included financial indicators, activity reports, upcoming projects and so on.

Each department was given the task of selecting a volunteer to sit at these meetings. The process of selecting a volunteer was simple. A special meeting was held in each department, the president's exchange concept was explained and the department directors asked for a volunteer to attend the monthly meetings with the president. If more than one person volunteered, straws were drawn to select the winner (or loser, depending on your point of view). There was no input or control on the part of management about who was selected. Looking back on the first several meetings, it became obvious that the employees did an excellent job in selecting their volunteers. There was a good mix of outspoken negative employees, some middle-of-the-road employees and some highly supportive employees. The interchange between the employees became quite constructive as these meetings progressed.

Finally, I implemented a suggestion box for employee ideas to come directly to the president and a bonus program which gave the employee with the best annual suggestion $500, an extra week's vacation and a special parking space for a year.

DO THE COOKS EAT IN THEIR KITCHEN?

Our second approach for gaining insights into employee perceptions came from an assembly meeting suggestion. A laboratory employee stood up during a question and answer period and made a profound suggestion. She said, "Why don't you conduct the same market survey among hospital employees as you are doing in the community?" To illustrate her point, she continued, "Sometimes cooks don't eat in their own kitchens because the food is so bad. Management should know how we employees feel about the quality of our own patient care."

My immediate reaction was, why hadn't I thought of that? Who better than the employees providing the patient care and services are able to form judgments about quality? They are certainly better equipped to judge the quality of care than most customers. So our market research firm was commissioned to conduct a random sample survey of employees, using the same questionnaire used in the community.

A random sample of 200 employees was needed to produce a confidence interval of plus or minus 5 percent for the results. It was critical to obtain the full cooperation of our employee group. The approach to gain that cooperation was to send a letter to the employees announcing that the suggestion had been made by a fellow employee to conduct a survey among employees and that the hospital had accepted that recommendation. The letter noted that 200 employees would have to participate in order to make the study valid. Employees were guaranteed anonymity by eliminating all of the demographic questions which might identify them and promising to share the results with all employees.

To guarantee anonymity, the listing of employees used by the market research firm was obtained in a unique way. On paycheck day, a sign-up sheet for employee phone numbers was posted. As the employees picked up their checks, they wrote down their current phone number but not their name. This list of 650 phone numbers was subsequently given to the market research firm. From this list the market research firm randomly selected 200 numbers for a survey. Only one employee declined to participate in the survey out of 200 who were called. The information gained from the survey, plus the direct personal insights gained from the assembly meetings, president's exchange and suggestion box, was extremely important in identifying our strengths and weaknesses and in developing strategies to move ahead.

<u>ASSESSING MANAGEMENT</u>

Downsizing management was discussed in chapter 2. As demanding and difficult as that task was, an even greater task came next—assessing the capability of the management staff that remained after downsizing. The term "management" included vice presidents and department directors. Department directors included the group of nursing managers referred to as head nurses by most hospitals.

In a turnaround the CEO should personally make the assessment of vice presidents and department directors. That is not to say that the vice presidents should have no input in evaluating department directors. However, in a turnaround it should be recognized that individuals at both the vice president level and the department director level may have contributed to the hospital's decline. To think that those same vice presidents could be entirely objective about their department directors' capabilities is unrealistic. The approach utilized at Beloit Memorial Hospital was to have the CEO do most of the critical evaluation of vice presidents and department directors. Downsizing the management organization took place three months after I started. The evaluations of management took place during the six months following the downsizing decisions.

A number of sources were utilized to make this assessment. Physician focus groups and the employee survey helped identify some weak management performers. In terms of objective data, performance indicators were reviewed for each department. This included a review of activity increases and decreases, utilization of manpower resources and utilization of financial resources. In other words, was a department's activity increasing, decreasing or

staying the same? Some departments, such as physical medicine, had experienced major increases in activity during the
past several years, even though the rest of the hospital's business had declined markedly. Activity gains were due in large
part to an extremely competent department director who
had earned the confidence of the physicians and the community. On the other hand, some departments were clearly
in decline as a result of poor leadership.

Qualitative and subjective judgments were part of the
management assessment also. For example, I did not feel the
hospital was as clean as it should be and I blamed that lack
of cleanliness on the leadership of the housekeeping department. The food was not very good either. It was easy to
learn this from talking to the patients and from eating in the
cafeteria. The fact that the food was poor was a reflection
on the leadership of the dietary department.

Assessment of the chemistry between the CEO, vice
presidents and department directors also played a part in the
assessment. As any experienced executive knows, you can
get along and work with some people and not others. This
does not necessarily mean that the "others" are incompetent. It merely means that the personalities and management styles may be incompatible. I relied on interviewing
skills to help determine who was going to stay and who was
not. As a rule of thumb, if there was someone so unacceptable in performance or attitude that I knew I would never
have hired him if I were interviewing for a vacant position,
then that person was not going to be acceptable to continue
his current position.

The integration of all assessments and evaluations led to
a decision that one half of the management staff of Beloit
Memorial Hospital needed to be replaced. Two of the four
vice presidents were replaced and twelve department directors replaced. In the interim, everyone pulled together and
made sure that the meals got out, the floors were cleaned
and the sick people well cared for. I cannot stress enough
that it is the CEO's responsibility and obligation to make
those difficult management replacement decisions. If he

does not, he is putting himself and his organization at risk since the burden of turning the organization around rests primarily with management.

LESSONS OF HINDSIGHT

As part of our management assessment and subsequent replacement decisions I learned that an organization can absorb far more management changes than I thought possible. It took approximately eighteen months to separate and recruit replacements for vice presidents and department directors who clearly did not meet my standards. That timetable was relatively slow since I was not convinced the organization could take a higher rate of management replacement. In hindsight, I could have made the changes in half the time. The day-to-day work of the institution went on, even when the management positions were vacant during recruiting. In some cases, it went better with the weak managers gone. It would have been better to separate everyone in a year or less, recruit their replacements and get on with it.

CHAPTER EIGHT

Symbols, Symbols, Symbols

THE USE OF BOLD symbols is very important to a successful hospital turnaround. Symbols can be effectively used by the CEO to send strong signals to the staff, physicians, board and community that progressive change is in the air. Symbolic messages can range from a "who's in charge" symbol to more subtle changes in the corporate culture. Symbols were very important during the first-year diagnosis and crisis management stages of Beloit Memorial Hospital's turnaround. They attracted attention, created controversy and generally confirmed that change was taking place. Things were so bad anyway I assumed change in itself was a positive force. I was almost right.

I once heard a well-known hospital CEO describe the "lobby painting" style of management. He encouraged new CEOs to paint the lobby of their new hospital immediately upon arrival. This symbolic gesture would supposedly let everyone know that change is imminent and positive. Use of symbols described in this chapter is an expanded version of "lobby painting."

In a turnaround, emotions are strained. Groups most closely involved with the hospital will be watching for positive and negative changes. They watch harder for negative ones. Creating positive impressions through the use of symbols is an important psychological aspect of the turnaround process. It is simply not enough to do the right things. People have to know that you are doing the right things and understand them. The use of symbols like those described here can help enormously in communicating the positive aspects of change.

POLISH THOSE SHOES

Perhaps the most immediate positive symbol that a new CEO can send employees is that he is listening. There are bound to be tremendous frustrations among employees when the leadership changes in a deteriorating hospital. Upon my arrival in Beloit, employees said that their biggest frustration was that they simply did not know what was going on. Being accessible and listening to employees during the early months is an excellent symbolic gesture. Creating new forms of communication like the assembly meetings, president's exchange and suggestion box gave substance to my listening approach.

Making the new CEO's personal standards immediately observable is another symbolic opportunity. Improving the appearance of employees and setting high dress code standards is one way to accomplish this. We have all seen the "St. Elsewhere" look on TV. Some hospitals are the living epitome of this look. Sending a few employees home to press their uniforms or polish their shoes will immediately become known throughout the hospital and is an excellent way to send the employees signals that staff appearance is important. One day I sent a dietary employee home to change his pants and shoes. The next day everyone in the dietary department could have passed a marine drill sergeant's inspection.

Another important symbolic gesture for employees is an immediate response to small problems. Walking through our intensive care unit at 2 a.m. one morning I noticed the ward clerk trying to write laboratory requisitions in the dark. When queried, she indicated that the previous administration had requested that the lights be kept off so as not to disturb the patients. An excellent idea. No one thought of the effect it would have on the working staff, however. An immediate fix was put in place the next day. Small, focused lights were installed so the ward clerk work area would be illuminated, but there would not be enough light to disturb the patients. Fixing some of these "irritaters" can go a long way in establishing that there is a new leader and that the hospital environment is going to improve.

Another way to make an immediate positive impression on employees is to improve the food and the parking situation. It's safe to say that no CEO ever fully satisfies his staff on these two issues. However, if he can make some visible improvements immediately after his arrival, it will send a clear and meaningful signal to the staff that those two important issues are being attended to. Our dietary department was not serving a hot breakfast to either patients or employees. That was quickly changed. Patients and employees alike appreciated having eggs and bacon instead of doughnuts and cold cereal.

Creating opportunities for after work social events can also be an effective symbol for employees. This may be particularly hard to do when a hospital is going through troubled times, yet the effort is well worth it. In my third month at Beloit Memorial Hospital I challenged the medical staff to a management vs. physician baseball game right in the midst of an employee layoff. Over 300 employees showed up to watch the medical staff destroy the management team by a score of 34–2. The game went a long way to ease the tension of the employee layoffs and gave the staff an opportunity to see the management and physicians in a social context.

END OF THE ART GALLERY

The lobby is a wonderful place to make some symbolic changes that will be immediately noticed not only by the employees and physicians, but by the community as well. I definitely subscribe to the "paint the lobby" theory. Beyond painting there are other changes which can also be utilized to communicate symbolically with the public. Some of mine were better received than others.

One change earned some immediate excellent responses from the community but made our volunteers mad as hell. The change was replacing the volunteers on the hospital's reception desk with full-time paid receptionists. Our hospital's reception area, like many around the country, was staffed by volunteers who only occasionally worked at the hospital. Their unfamiliarity with the hospital's services and building layout caused a great deal of confusion for visitors. Additionally, the use of volunteers led to inconsistent customer greeting practices and attitudes. Full-time receptionists were hired. This displaced volunteers into other activities. There is no doubt that this caused a backlash among the volunteers who dearly loved their front desk assignment. For a time I thought all 400 volunteers were going to picket the hospital in protest. Employee pickets were bad enough. The prospect of volunteer pickets could shatter the confidence of even the most aggressive CEO. I was saved only because the change was a tremendous improvement for the public and patients.

Another positive change a new CEO can make is to improve the art work in the public areas of the hospital. Many hospitals have become quasi-art galleries for local artists. Although this sometimes works well, in our hospital it had created a negative image. People bought the "good" paintings almost immediately. The less desirable paintings hung around for months and years. Our walls were covered with a hodge-podge of local art bearing price tags. The most controversial move I made during my first several weeks was to remove the local artwork and replace it with a bright eclectic collection of framed posters from around the country. It improved the overall appearance of the building but inspired the local artists to burn me in effigy on the high school football field. Since this program was run by the volunteers, it gave them another reason to be up in arms. It's a good thing I don't go to cocktail parties. I was the subject of roastings at Beloit's parties for months.

The grounds are another area to make some immediate symbolic points. If they have been neglected, the CEO can insist on improvements which make a much more positive first impression on patients and visitors. Additionally, the judicious use of paint and wallpaper throughout the building can do a great deal to improve the physical environment of the facility without costing a great deal of money. The new CEO should remember that the physical environment of the building and grounds is a reflection of his own standards and values. If it is a sloppy looking unprofessional environment, there is no one to blame but himself. There are risks to making improvements, however. I learned this the hard way when I received an angry letter from a local citizen who gave me a written tongue lashing for wasting money on wood chips around our trees and walkways. Writing a letter letting this whistle blower know that a local contractor had donated the wood chips made my day.

Outside signs are another good area to make a positive symbolic statement to the community. Have you ever had the experience of trying to read one inch letters on parking signs from your car at a distance of fifty or sixty feet? It is nearly impossible, as I found when I arrived for my first day of work and tried to locate the employee parking lot. Improving the signs and making them readable will generate some immediate positive feedback from the customers who use your facility. The opportunity should not be missed.

TERMINATIONS ARE SYMBOLS TOO

There were two kinds of unusual terminations which had major symbolic implications during the early months of our turnaround. Both involved individuals who technically were not employed by the hospital.

The first terminations involved physicians working in our emergency room. Within a month of my arrival two physicians were terminated. One physician had a habit of pursuing his love life while on duty and leaving the emergency room uncovered. Another physician left the emergency room before his replacement reported for duty, leaving the emergency room briefly with no attending physician. The firing of these physicians by the hospital sent an immediate signal to our contract firm that such unprofessional conduct was no longer acceptable. More importantly it sent a signal to the hospital employees that physicians were going to be held accountable to a newer and higher set of standards than they had been in the past.

Before the first year was completed, other attending physicians whose professional behavior had been less than acceptable had also been disciplined. I even suspended a physician over a clinical response problem. That had never happened before. Not surprisingly, physician behavior began to improve. There was less acting up and more attention to clinical practice by the physicians who had tended to neglect these responsibilities. I should add that the great majority of physicians were excellent in terms of attitude and clinical quality. However, the laissez faire attitude of management had let a few bad boys get away with behavior and clinical problems. These boys quickly found out that their behavior would no longer be tolerated.

The second unusual terminations involved volunteers. Several volunteers were fired for attitude problems, an unheard of occurrence at our hospital and I suspect at most others. The great majority of volunteers in our hospital were dedicated individuals. A few, however, saw as their mission the critique of changes being made at the hospital. Sometimes they went too far. One volunteer who didn't like the color of the new lobby carpet began exclaiming to all visitors who would listen that hospital rates were going to increase because of the new carpet. A few others felt that breaking patient confidentiality and being rude was acceptable since they were volunteers, not paid employees. Four volunteers were dismissed for attitude issues and several others given stern warnings during the first year.

At first, these actions were seen as overly harsh. Some nasty things were said about that new SOB who had the gall to fire someone who worked for free. However, when the dust settled the volunteers themselves became aware of a new sense of pride in being seen as the equal of our employees in status, even if it meant equal for discipline too. After a few more months the volunteers themselves effectively dealt with problem individuals in their own ranks. I never had to say another word about the need for everyone associated with the hospital to display a positive attitude, whether they worked for free or not.

PHYSICIAN AMENITIES ARE IMPORTANT

Some hospital CEOs believe that one of their most important roles is making physicians' lives as miserable as possible, particularly when it comes to amenities. Those executives would not succeed in a turnaround. Physicians need to be seen as working partners, not antagonists. Treating them well is a prerequisite of a successful turnaround.

Physicians represent many opportunities to make early symbolic moves. Attention to some of their small problems will be immediately noticed. If their parking spaces aren't close enough to the building, get them closer ones. If there are not enough, expand the parking lot. I doubled the size of the physician parking lot shortly after I arrived. This was the only change I made which drew absolutely no negative comments from physicians. Of course, the employees who lost their spaces near the building reacted predictably by whining about walking another twenty feet.

Another important symbolic move which can be made to physicians is improving the food for staff meetings. I don't mean to sound cynical. However, it has been my experience that if excellent meals are provided for physician meetings, attendance will be far greater than if you provide inferior meals or none at all. We go out of our way at our hospital to be sure that physicians are well treated with reference to the amenities and meals at their meetings. It definitely improved attendance at our staff meetings. I also secretly hoped they would all gain enough weight so management could beat them in softball. It didn't work, however.

Communicating with physicians, as with employees, is an important symbolic gesture. Listening to physician needs early in the turnaround is very important. Acting on their needs, if financially feasible, will go a long way to establishing credibility and trust between the hospital's management and physicians. Carrying that one step further, communicating the facts of the turnaround situation to physicians can also be very helpful.

I made a commitment upon my arrival at Beloit Memorial Hospital to give the medical staff the exact same information on a monthly basis as was provided to the board. This meant they received financial performance data, activity projections and a summary of the key projects and activities which were facing the hospital. This open communication brought management and physicians closer together. Taking physicians into management's confidence can work to their advantage. The confidential way our physicians treated their advance knowledge of our layoffs confirmed the success of this approach.

I don't mean to give the reader the impression that Beloit Memorial Hospital is a Mecca for physician/management relations. Far from it. I had a number of very vocal critics. No matter what changes were made, these critics found fault. Unlike some CEOs who get tied in knots by the "lunatic fringe" physician dictators, I ignored them. It drove them crazy that no matter how hard they tried, I never took them on in public. In private was another matter.

THE BUCK STOPS WHERE?

The board can also benefit from symbols from the CEO. If the previous CEO made a practice of bringing a passel of subordinates to board meetings, then the first symbolic move I suggest is the discontinuance of this practice. During a turnaround, the board must see its CEO as the hospital leader. Bringing subordinates to board meetings and having them make presentations dilutes the perception of leadership. I quickly discontinued my predecessor's practice of bringing an assistant to board meetings and made it clear to the board I did not expect them to communicate with my subordinates on hospital business.

Secondly, the CEO can quickly earn the respect of his board by organizing the meetings and streamlining them. If the board is in the habit of reading minutes during meetings and always utilizing a rigid agenda, the CEO and chairman should make improvements. Minutes should be distributed prior to the meeting and reviewed carefully by board members at home. It is a waste of time to read minutes. It puts everybody to sleep. If any comments are necessary, they should be questions or exceptions. With reference to the agenda, the CEO should work with the board chairman to create agendas which are tailored to the meetings, not the other way around. Many times board meetings are so structured that the routine items come first, like review of the financial statements, and the really important items for discussion come so much later in the meeting that people are either falling asleep or their attention is severely distracted. Beloit adopted changes in the board meeting format soon after my arrival. Minutes were no longer read, and agendas were changed to put the most important items first. Attendance at board meetings and the quality of discussion improved dramatically.

Lastly, the CEO should establish with the board that he is in charge of the operation of the hospital. This can be effectively done by insisting that board members refer complaints, inquiries from the press, vendor issues, etc., to the CEO for follow up. The CEO then has the obligation to follow up and get back to the board member who brought the matter to his attention in the first place.

BE FELT IN THE COMMUNITY, NOT HEARD

In a turnaround, CEOs should avoid the practice of becoming community statesmen, visible on community boards, the Rotary, etc. Although these may be perfectly reasonable activities under normal circumstances, it will divert the CEO's attention from the turnaround without producing any positive results for the hospital. The tendency to be a joiner should be avoided in favor of focusing on the job. I learned that lesson the hard way. I joined the Rotary and the board of directors of a community service agency soon after my arrival in Beloit. My efforts, however, were so focused on the hospital that I missed nearly all of the Rotary lunches and board meetings. Soon I was thrown out of both organizations which was embarrassing, to say the least. It left a lasting impression that I was not really needed in those organizations. Nor was my participation contributing anything to turning around the hospital.

The same thing can be said for participating in local, state or national hospital associations. While these activities may be personally rewarding and interesting, they do nothing to help turnaround a troubled hospital. An outside man is not what is needed during a turnaround.

Hospital CEOs would do well to evaluate the "inside oriented trend" for corporate CEOs. Changes in the leadership orientation of General Electric are a good illustration. GE's chairman during the 1970s, Reginald Jones, saw himself as a civic leader and corporate statesman. His role as a public figure, speaker and consultant to presidents kept him so busy he left the running of the company to a huge corporate staff. All the while GE's corporate performance was lackluster. His successor, John Welch, sits on no corporate boards other than GE, makes few speeches and rarely visits Washington. Indeed, he leads GE. Gone are the huge corporate staff, tens of thousands of white collar workers and the stodgy image and mediocre performance. Today's GE is more profitable and dynamic. Its success is at least partly due to a leader who sees himself as an inside man rather than an outside statesman.

Limiting the access of the press can also be a constructive move during a turnaround. It is safe to say that the CEO will be undertaking some difficult and sometimes controversial activities like layoffs, management changes and so on. Talking about them in the press will not do the organization any good in my judgment. My recommendation is to say very little if anything during the early turnaround stages. If good things are happening at the hospital, they should be saved for later publication. If the hospital tries to negate the effect of bad publicity caused by layoffs and firings by using "good" news stories, you can be assured the good news stories will get less attention than glamorous stories like layoffs.

Another important symbolic gesture for the community is to level with community leaders about the circumstances of the hospital. Early in my tenure at Beloit Memorial Hospital I invited community leaders to attend briefings which spelled out the difficult situation the hospital was in. They appreciated the honesty and directness of those meetings. It also laid the groundwork for those community leaders to be future advocates of the hospital when the problems had been resolved. Communicating effectively with community leaders is a much more productive activity than trying to tell your story to the newspaper. Newspapers are in business to sell papers and make a profit. Community leaders, on the other hand, have a vested interest in their hospital and will likely respond very positively to being taken into your confidence.

LESSONS OF HINDSIGHT

Without question the best symbolic decision made early in our turnaround was hiring receptionists for the lobby desk. Although the displaced volunteers were temporarily upset, even they could not argue that the public and our customers were better served with permanent receptionists.

On the other hand, the handling of the local artists' paintings was poorly done and caused hard feelings. When the artists found out that the hospital was planning to discontinue the selling of local work, they got mad and immediately removed all of their paintings. The local newspaper even ran an editorial scolding me as an "elitist." It took nearly a month to place new posters on the walls, and in the meantime the hospital walls looked barren and sterile. That made everyone involved even madder.

CHAPTER NINE

Chiseling the Strategic Slate

NEAR THE END of year one the information gathering projects were completed. While I had focused internally on crisis management, a series of research projects, focus groups, personal interviews and community surveys was underway. The news was not encouraging.

Organizing the various sources of input into an overall assessment was the next step in our turnaround. It required taking a step back and collating the numerous sources of input to take a hard and objective look at ourselves. It was a necessary step in planning what to do next. The crisis management steps were working. Now it was time to make some judgments about what caused the hospital's decline and what steps would be necessary for recovery.

COMMUNITY MARKET RESEARCH FINDINGS

The charge to our market research firm was threefold. Find out how many people were leaving Beloit for hospital care; find out why they were leaving; and find out if current patients were satisfied with hospital services. The most dramatic and depressing finding of our community research was that 34 percent of local residents were out-migrating for hospital services. This one fact put into perspective why hospital activity had declined so precipitously. Beloit residents had not suddenly gotten healthier. Instead, those needing hospital care had decided that they were better off traveling to competing hospitals. This, more than any other factor, explained our dramatic decline in inpatient business. Along with the overall out-migration figures, it was also discovered where our residents were going.

In constructing the community study, it was hypothesized that our biggest hospital competitor was a similar community hospital about 10 miles away. This hospital was easily accessible to Beloit residents, and offered services similar to Beloit Memorial Hospital's. Much to our surprise, the data showed this hospital was not our key competitor. Instead, Beloit residents were traveling approximately 20 miles to the three tertiary hospitals located in a nearby major metropolitan area. Each of these hospitals had a strong reputation and a wider range of primary and tertiary services than Beloit Memorial Hospital. Both the telephone surveys and the focus group findings confirmed that Beloit Memorial Hospital had a lot to worry about. Its community had lost confidence. Horror stories about the hospital were recent and much repeated. The hospital's reputation was at rock bottom.

The community surveys identified five specific areas of dissatisfaction with Beloit Memorial Hospital. This answered the second question of why people were leaving the community for hospital services. Areas of dissatisfaction were:

1. *Emergency Room*—Research showed tremendous dissatisfaction with the quality and attitude of the physicians in the emergency room. Emergency physician services were provided by a large outside contract group. It was clear that the community was not responding well to these physicians.

2. *Specialists*—Research also confirmed that people were leaving the community because of the unavailability of certain medical specialists. Cardiology, neurology, psychiatry and oncology were mentioned prominently as reasons for out-migration.

3. *Low Tech Image*—It became clear from the community research that Beloit residents perceived their hospital as low tech. Residents felt it necessary to travel to nearby tertiary hospitals to get the best available in medical technology. They were right.

4. *Convenience Services*—Residents were also out-migrating because the hospital lacked convenience services. Most notably absent was a day surgery facility in Beloit. All of the three nearby tertiary hospitals offered day surgery programs which attracted Beloit residents.

5. *Attitude and Responsiveness*—Community residents blamed hospital management for not responding to their wants and needs. There was also a clear and consistent message from the community that the attitude of hospital employees was poor and unresponsive to patient needs. The bottom line on this issue was that the community felt the hospital was not listening.

As far as the third market research question, satisfaction levels of existing customers, the news was also bad. Only 55 percent of the Beloit community preferred Beloit Memorial Hospital as their hospital of choice. This was an astoundingly low level for a one hospital community, according to our market research firm. Even with the advantage of no local competition, only half the community preferred Beloit as their hospital of choice.

It wasn't all bad news, however. The initial survey confirmed that maternity services and the physical therapy department were well perceived in the community. It was also learned that the majority of Beloit residents who were out-migrating might be willing to reconsider and come back to their local hospital if changes were made. These were small but encouraging glimmers of hope.

PHYSICIAN FINDINGS

Findings of the physician focus groups and interviews by management were consistent with the community market research, but they also provided additional insights. Physicians identified maternity service and sub-specialty physicians in the area of vascular surgery and gastrointestinal disease as major clinical strengths. At the same time, physicians identified emergency room physicians and the absence of neurology, oncology and cardiology services as medical weaknesses. Physicians pinpointed weaknesses in employee morale and nursing skills. They also speculated that hospital departments such as education and laboratory needed better leadership.

Physician interviews identified a schism between the specialists in the community's large sub-specialty clinic and family practitioners who were independent of the clinic. Opinions varied among physicians about how severe this schism actually was; however, tensions between the two groups were leading to a higher than desired level of out-migration. As an example, when a family practitioner did not like the clinic's only cardiologist, he simply referred all his cardiology patients out of town. This was one of the reasons that three-fourths of the cardiology business was leaving town.

Physician focus groups helped identify the need for better communication between the hospital management and physicians as a prerequisite for more effective working relationships. Physicians also identified several good ideas, like having a patient ombudsman to help resolve patient problems. They seized the opportunity to put in requests for better parking spaces, a private lounge, and longer food service hours.

EMPLOYEE FINDINGS

The employee survey results represented both good news and bad news. The survey was conducted near the end of year one, after most of the internal crisis management decisions had been implemented. The good news was that employees had a much higher opinion of the quality of care than the community. Employees are a leading indicator of community perceptions. If the quality of care is improving, hospital employees will know about it before the community. On the other hand, if care is deteriorating, employees recognize it before the general community. As one midwestern hospital learned the hard way, the hospital staff can either be your biggest help or your biggest hindrance in turning around a negative image. That hospital discovered its own nurses recommending that newcomers to the community use another hospital because their hospital was understaffed. We found quite the opposite. Our staff seemed to have a much higher level of confidence in the quality of care than the community.

The surveys also confirmed that our employees were responding well to the new hospital leadership approaches. This was particularly true with our nursing department. Many good ideas came from the staff during the critical first year. For example, RNs had recommended that the hospital implement minimum continuing education standards for all RNs in order to maintain their status as full-time employees. They recommended that each RN be required to take at least 12 hours of continuing education per year, and that if 12 hours were not achieved they be removed from the payroll. Can you imagine that? If that suggestion had come from top management it probably would have been labeled communism. On the other hand, coming from the staff it appeared to be a genuine and sincere effort at upgrading the quality of clinical skills at the bedside.

All in all, the positive attitude and responsiveness of our employees to change was encouraging. Their flexibility and commitment to improving the hospital's image played a major role in subsequent successes.

SWOT: Getting it all together

When taken in their entirety, the various input gathering sources enabled the hospital to create a comprehensive listing of strengths, weaknesses, opportunities and threats: SWOT. Here is what our SWOT assessment yielded.

1. *Strengths*—The following were identified as major hospital strengths:

   - Solo Hospital: Being the only hospital in town should give us a definite competitive advantage.

   - Medical Specialties: Vascular surgery, maternity and gastroenterology were judged to be excellent.

   - Physical Medicine: This department was the fastest growing and highest quality department in the hospital.

   - Physician/Administrative Relations: These were excellent. The CEO was definitely in the honeymoon phase.

   - Low Cost: Comparative data indicated that Beloit Memorial Hospital was among the lowest cost hospitals in the surrounding area.

2. *Weaknesses*—The following represented major hospital weaknesses:

   - Emergency Room Physician Quality: The single greatest medical deficit was physician practice in the emergency room, both in attitude and clinical performance.

   - Medical Specialty Voids: Absence of local physician specialists was a major weakness, especially in the areas of neurology, cardiology, oncology and urology.

   - Low Image: Only 55 percent of our community perceived Beloit as their hospital of choice.

   - Nursing Quality and Image: Both the community and medical staff identified the quality of nursing skills and morale as a major weakness.

- Financial Weakness: The hospital's huge past operating losses and projected future losses put it at risk for defaulting on its loan obligations if activity declines continued.

- Community Relations: The absence of an organized and effective community relations program was clearly a hospital weakness.

3. *Opportunities*—The following areas were seen as opportunities to improve the hospital's competitive position:

- Promote Medical Strengths: Maternity service represented the best perceived service in the community. It represented an opportunity to promote the hospital and medical staff jointly.

- New Medical Specialists: The recruitment of desired medical specialists represented a major opportunity to reverse medical out-migration pattern.

- Affiliation with Tertiary Hospital: The affiliation with a major tertiary hospital represented an opportunity to improve the hospital's image and obtain needed specialty coverage.

- Convenience Service: Implementation of more convenience oriented services, particularly day surgery services, was a major opportunity to reduce out-migration.

- Specialty Development: Development and promotion of already highly perceived medical services such as the vascular service was seen as an opportunity to promote existing medical strengths.

4. *Threats*—The following represented major threats to the hospital's survival:

- Census Declines: Census decline trends for the past six years were alarming. If they continued through 1985, the hospital census would decline to approximately 70 inpatients per day. At that point, the hospital would not be able to cover fixed expenses and would have to file for bankruptcy.

- Tertiary Hospital Competition: The three tertiary hospitals previously mentioned in the major metropolitan area a short distance away represented major competitive threats.

- HMO and PPO Competition: HMOs and PPOs were being developed by nearby tertiary hospitals for marketing in the Beloit area. Since Beloit had neither HMOs nor PPOs to offer, these competitive initiatives represented a major threat.

- Surgi-Center Construction: At the time the SWOT assessment was completed, two for-profit surgi-center applications had been filed for the Beloit area. These projects represented a major threat to existing surgery business.

- Work Force Downsizing: The necessity to downsize the employee work force to preserve financial stability represented a major continuing threat to the already low employee morale.

- Management Turnover: Management turnover due to downsizing of the management staff and separation of managers judged not compatible with the new leadership represented a major stability problem.

ENTER THE STRATEGIC SLATE

Many more issues faced Beloit Memorial Hospital than were identified in our SWOT assessment. The lists were endless. The SWOT assessment forced us to focus on the most important issues. SWOT challenged our ability to make early decisions about what was important and what was not important. It also helped us to avoid making bold moves in areas that were weak. Mistakes like promoting a weak service such as the emergency room were avoided. As more than one marketing consultant has said, the worst thing that you can do with a weak product is to push it. More people will try it and find out how bad it really is. Finally, the SWOT assessment enabled us to complete our short term turnaround plans, the "strategic slate."

What is a strategic slate? It is a limited set of measurable and prioritized objectives which need to be accomplished to ensure survival. The strategic slate gave us the focus necessary to concentrate on what was important, and was the planning vehicle for achieving a unified effort to save our hospital. Lastly, the strategic slate gave the hospital management and board the end points which, when achieved, would be grounds for celebration. At least we hoped there would be cause for celebration.

The strategic slate of Beloit Memorial Hospital was completed by myself and the four vice presidents, with assistance from our marketing consultants. The process required several full day meetings with Terry Rynne acting as a moderator. The top management group provided the energy, creativity and decisions needed to focus on the key areas which would lead to survival. Terry provided the coaching and played the role of devil's advocate if we strayed from focusing on measurable goals.

The strategic slate development process was to use the SWOT assessment to identify the goals first. Then definitive measures of success were formulated. Detailed implementation plans to achieve the desired goals were the last step.

WHAT A STRATEGIC SLATE IS NOT

It is important to note what a strategic slate is not. The strategic slate is not an endless list of fuzzy goals. It is not a wish list of things that a management is going to try to accomplish. It is not a long list with imprecise statements like "improving morale" or "reducing costs." It is not a document produced by an outside consultant, destined to be stuck in a drawer only to emerge when the JCAH demands evidence of institutional planning.

What is it then? It is a short list of measurable targets created by the people who have to achieve those targets. It is a page or two long that becomes smudged with finger prints and perhaps an occasional tear or two, because it is referred to so often. It is a concise document which focuses the management's efforts on those tasks which make the difference between the hospital's life or death. And, it is a document with which the board can measure objectively the effectiveness of its management.

BELOIT MEMORIAL HOSPITAL'S STRATEGIC SLATE

Beloit Memorial Hospital's strategic slate included six objectives. The achievement of each of the six objectives was necessary to insure the hospital's survival. The objectives were:

1. *Emergency Medicine Physicians*
   The first goal was the recruitment of four emergency medicine residency trained physicians. If accomplished, Beloit Memorial Hospital would become the first hospital in Wisconsin to have its emergency room staffed exclusively with emergency medicine, residency trained physicians.

2. *Technology Update*
   Evaluation of each clinical department's equipment and commitment of $1.5 million to upgrade the equipment became our second goal.

3. *Day Surgery*
   Designing, building and promoting a new day surgery unit became our third goal.

4. *Medical Specialists*
   Recruiting a neurologist, cardiologist and oncologist in conjunction with the community's clinic and creation of an affiliation partnership with a major tertiary hospital became goal number four.

5. *Financial Stability*
   Bringing the hospital back into the black from recent periods of major operating losses became goal number five.

6. *Attitude and Responsiveness*
   Creating an extremely responsive customer service organization and producing a statistically significant improve-

ment in community attitudes as measured by market research became our sixth goal.

WHO DOES WHAT?

One important aspect of succeeding with a strategic slate is accountability. After the six goals were agreed upon by management and approved by the board, they were assigned to the top management staff. The vice president of professional services was assigned the emergency physician recruitment goal. The vice president of support services took on the technology upgrade goal. The vice president of nursing assumed responsibility to develop a day surgery facility. The vice president of finance was assigned to implement strategies to return the hospital to profitability. I undertook the medical recruitment and employee attitude improvement goals. Our jobs were on the line. Success on strategic slate goals meant survival for the hospital, and for us as management. Failure guaranteed at the very least that we would lose our jobs, and maybe even our hospital.

Beloit Memorial Hospital's strategic slate was finalized at the end of year one. Year two was established as the period to achieve those six goals. The strategic slate became our focus, our passion and our cause for celebration one year later.

TAKING STOCK

At the end of year one, things were looking up. The projected loss of $500,000 was reversed and the hospital made a modest profit of $162,000. The crisis management strategies had worked, and we had a plan to correct the problems which had caused the hospital's decline.

It was a tough year, but two things stick in my mind about its passing. First, the board generously rewarded my performance with an excellent raise. They were clearly pleased, and relieved. Second, I began getting calls from executive search firms to take on bigger hospitals in need of a turnaround. I could hardly believe that one year's work could attract so much attention, but the offers were proof that other hospitals were anxious to have a turnaround "expert."

Although I never followed up on the recruitment calls, I must admit that receiving them gave me a sense of comfort. It was great to know that if something happened in Beloit other hospitals were clamoring for CEOs with turnaround experience. That knowledge gave me the confidence to plunge ahead in Beloit doing things my way. The absence of a "golden parachute" became less and less important with each head-hunter call. Perhaps the courage was artificial, but at the start of year two I was ready to take it wherever I could find it.

LESSONS OF HINDSIGHT

When CEOs turn over, whether a turnaround is necessary or not, there is an inclination to do a long-range plan. In a turnaround, this long range review should be avoided. You can spend $150,000 and take a year to create or update a long-range plan, using outside consultants. In the meantime the hospital might go bankrupt. In the short run, survival is the most important thing. First find out what needs to be done to survive and do it. Our use of a strategic slate kept us focused on several objectives. That focus enabled us to succeed.

In hindsight, one more goal should have been added to the slate. Goal number seven would have been, "Remember to have fun and keep your sense of humor when accomplishing goals one through six."

PART III

YEAR TWO: TREATMENT

Memorable Moment #3:
"I purchased a bottle of Dom Perignon at
the restaurant and had it placed in a
doggie bag for a celebration on the way
home. As the chartered plane taxied to the
runway, the champagne was uncorked,
and a toast was offered to our first big
success."

CHAPTER TEN

Start at the Top

AT THE BEGINNING of year two, Beloit Memorial Hospital had a clear sense of direction and purpose. Carrying out our strategic slate presented major management challenges. While a number of positions were eliminated when the management organization was downsized, there were major weaknesses in the remaining management group. As year two began, I decided to begin rebuilding the management staff by starting at the top and working down.

One-half of the management staff of Beloit Memorial Hospital was replaced. Two of the four vice presidents were replaced and 12 of the 24 department directors replaced. Recruitment of the new vice presidents and department directors took 18 months. A combination of approaches was used to recruit the new managers. They included personal contacts, advertising and executive search firms. Advertising and personal contacts were the primary approaches.

Replacing half of a management staff is a formidable task in any organization. There were times when I wondered if I was moving too fast. Hindsight proved that rather than moving too fast, I probably could have proceeded with the replacements on an even faster schedule. Even when

management jobs were unfilled following terminations, the
day-to-day work still went on largely because of our motivated work force. Taking our time and being extremely se-
lective in the recruitment process was the right approach in
the long run. But that strategy resulted in leaving some management positions unfilled for nearly a year. Replacing half
of a management staff may seem particularly aggressive. But
keep in mind that weak management led to the hospital's
decline in the first place. Luckily for me and Beloit Memorial Hospital, the half retained were extremely strong and responded well to new leadership.

Our hospital had four vice presidents. Two were capable and were retained. Vice President of Finance John Morgan had an excellent industry background prior to entering
the hospital industry several years earlier. His industry perspective, maturity and executive skills brought a fresh approach to the financial management of our hospital.
Nursing Vice President Vanetta Gerhardt was also retained.
She had a long track record of rising through the nursing
ranks and had an excellent sense of history and perspective
on the organization due to her three decades of service. I
was fortunate that two of the four vice presidents were
strong enough to be retained. In a turnaround there is need
for continuity at the top if at all possible. These two excellent executives provided the hospital with that needed continuity.

Our vice presidents of professional services and support services needed to be replaced. Their capabilities, attitudes and work ethic were inconsistent with the new
hospital leadership's direction. Both executives were separated with severance agreements and outplacement counseling services. The search process for replacements was begun
by formulating a new position description for vice presidents. Appendix B is a sample of the position description
utilized. Beyond defining position expectations, I identified
several personal characteristics that were very important in
the selection process. In a nutshell, I wanted executives who
were hungry for advancement and a risky career challenge.

Executives should not join an organization in need of a turnaround unless they are risk takers. Loyalty and flexibility were also key desired characteristics. Turnarounds test an individual's loyalty in a hundred different ways. The ability to be flexible and accept a variety of assignments is a must. Lastly, the ability to work long hours and roll up the shirt sleeves were desired work ethic characteristics. One of the separated vice presidents had demonstrated the opposite of this characteristic. He lived 60 miles from the hospital. His idea of a full day's work was a mere eight hours, including two hours of commuting time. He rarely spent more than six hours on the job. With that kind of top management example, it was no wonder that a poor work ethic permeated the middle management ranks.

I began building the new team with the recruitment of a vice president for professional services. This individual was going to lead the key clinical departments of the hospital, as shown in figure 3 (p. 24). Some of this division's department heads were being retained and were excellent managers. They needed a leader they could look up to and who could facilitate their professional development. There was also to be some department head recruitment in this division, since some managers were quite weak. Additionally, I planned to make the individual in this position my informal "No. 2." I needed someone I could trust and rely on to oversee the hospital in my absence.

For this critical position, I tapped an executive whose skills and capabilities were well known to me—Gregory Britton. I still recall calling him at 10 o'clock on an August evening at the close of what had been the worst day of my new job. Union representatives had picketed the hospital that morning, and the Maalox I had consumed for breakfast had done little to calm my stomach. Greg was an assistant administrator at my former hospital and I had known him for about 10 years. Greg had an interesting management background. He came up through the ranks to his former position of assistant administrator. He began his career as an occupational therapist and subsequently took on increasing responsibilities as director of rehabilitation, administrative assistant and assistant administrator. His experiences, particularly as a department head, gave him a perspective that was especially valuable in our turnaround setting.

I presented the career opportunity to Greg in a glamourous light. I told him that I had a position with an extremely high career risk, low pay and long hours. But I stressed the opportunity to really impact the fate of Beloit Memorial Hospital. I told him that if we failed, the management would all be out on the street. If, on the other hand, we succeeded in turning Beloit Memorial Hospital around, it would be due in large part to the efforts of the top management group. It was a career opportunity where an individual could make a difference to an organization's survival. After a few visits to Beloit, Greg agreed to join the hospital's management staff. His excellent leadership unquestionably made a big difference between success and failure during the turnaround.

Next, I turned my attention to recruiting a vice president of support services. That division needed to be developed from the ground up. There were several excellent department heads, but others clearly needed to be replaced. I wanted a real hands on executive in this position. Early in my career this division had been one of my first big assignments. I had learned the support services departments by getting my hands dirty in the housekeeping and dietary departments and by learning the intricacies of purchasing and central supply. It was a rewarding experience. I wanted to find someone who would approach the job from that perspective rather than a "big executive" perspective.

For this recruitment, I called CEOs that I had known during my career and asked for advice and referrals. Fortunately one of my CEO aquaintances in the Boston area knew just the executive to fit our needs. John Chioutsis, a young man finishing an administrative residency at the CEO's hospital, was looking for a permanent position. His background was extremely interesting. He had been a heart-lung machine operator for five years prior to deciding to go into hospital administration. His mixture of clinical background and newly acquired administrative experience through graduate school and an administrative residency was just the right combination for our hands-on vice president of support services opportunity. He was eager to learn administration from the ground up. John came into the organization with his shirt sleeves rolled up and hasn't stopped learning and contributing since.

All four vice presidents worked tirelessly to turn Beloit Memorial Hospital around. They were just the right combination of youth, maturity and experience. They put themselves into our organization and formed a team which ensured Beloit Memorial Hospital's recovery and success. The community owes them a tremendous debt of thanks. They saved the hospital.

ON TO THE DEPARTMENTS

Eleven new department directors were brought into the organization during the turnaround. Six of these positions became open because of terminations. The individuals occupying those positions were separated due to poor performance, poor attitude or both. Three more of the position openings were due to turnover. These individuals left the community in the early phases of the turnaround due to spouse relocation or dissatisfaction with the new management style. Two other positions opened due to retirement. The remaining position opened as a result of creating a new department director position in finance.

Seven departmental positions were filled through classified advertising. Two positions were filled through internal promotion. Two positions were filled by an executive search firm, and the remaining position was not filled because its duties were consolidated into the job of another department director.

Ten department directors were retained from the previous administration. There were some extremely capable leaders in that group. These individuals excelled in their re-spective departments almost in spite of bad leadership. They did not allow themselves to be dragged down either personally or professionally. They continued to strive for excellence and succeeded.

As with the vice president recruitments, department director recruitments were started by updating the department director job descriptions. A sample of the new position descriptions is provided in Appendix C. Beyond the job description requirements, several important personality characteristics were sought for our new middle managers. First, individuals who sought career advancements, rather than lateral moves, were desired. Individuals who were flexible in their attitudes and willing to accept unconventional assignments were given top priority.

Only individuals who felt comfortable with a hands on management style from above were sought. This was particularly important, since many hospital department directors operate semi-autonomously. Their assistant administrators or vice presidents do not really get into the details of the day-to-day operation. In our hospital, vice presidents were expected to become familiar with their departments and to practice a hands-on management approach. Department directors who felt comfortable and stimulated by this approach, rather than threatened by it, were needed.

Advertising proved to be the most successful approach in recruiting new department directors. Regional newspapers and professional journals were used with equal success in generating qualified candidates. Expenses were not spared in advertising. Large and attractive advertisements were used and generated a large number of candidates to choose from for each open position. For most positions, at least one hundred applications were received. Ten to twenty applicants were well qualified.

INTERVIEWS AND SHOW AND TELL

The vice presidents were responsible for recruitment of department directors in their divisions. They screened applicant's résumés and conducted telephone interviews with the most promising candidates. From the telephone interviews, top candidates were selected for on-site visits. The interview teams varied with the type of position. For the most part, they consisted of several vice presidents, several department directors, physicians (for clinical department director positions) and a community real estate agent.

Some hospitals balk at using physicians in the interview process for department directors. Our experiences with physicians were excellent. Enthusiastic physicians helped "sell" our hospital to prospective candidates. For first interviews, spouses were always invited, even though that is not common practice. By spending a few extra dollars on the initial interview, we usually made a positive impression on spouses. This helped recruit the individuals that we really wanted, since many hospitals skimp on spouse interviews. Spouses were courted every bit as much as the candidates themselves.

After the first series of interviews, usually one or two candidates stood out. Those candidates were invited back. The second interview was always sufficient to identify the candidate of choice. When the final candidate had been selected, an unusual last step was added to our selection process. In almost every case, site visits were made to the final candidate's hospital to observe firsthand evidence of their performance. For example, when hiring a new dietary director our vice president of support services made a site visit to the final candidate's hospital to sample the food and to talk with patients and employees about how good the food *really* was.

This approach was particularly helpful for service departments. Candidates can be excellent interviewees and still be lousy managers. Making site visits separated the big talkers from the people who really produced. Although this strategy is not frequently utilized by other hospitals, it has enabled us to recruit higher caliber department directors. It also gives prospective candidates strong confirmation about how interested we really are in results.

Executive search firms were used for two key department director positions. The director of human resources
position and the director of maternity services benefited
from national searches conducted by Quigley Associates of
Burr Ridge, Illinois. The human resources position was absolutely critical to our ongoing success. Since this position
reported directly to me and I was unable to devote the personal recruiting time the search deserved, I elected to use a
search firm. The director of maternity services position was
also extremely important. Our physicians and community
market research identified the maternity service as being
our strongest nursing department. The department deserved an excellent leader. Since there were no inhouse or
local candidates for the job, a search firm was used. Both
searches were conducted very competently, and the candidates presented were uniformly excellent.

To initiate these two searches, we worked with the
search consultant to update position descriptions and identify desired personal characteristics. Then the salary and
benefit package were agreed upon and the search consultant
began his task. Both searches took about six months. While
this may seem like a long time, we were very picky, and the
candidates and the managers ultimately recruited for these
positions were of such high caliber that the wait was well
worth it. The interview process for search firm candidates
was the same as for candidates identified through advertising programs and personal contacts. The search firm approach was far more expensive than doing it ourselves, but
it saved a great deal of time. Advertising is less expensive,
but takes more time. Individual circumstances dictate which
strategy is better.

Internal promotions were utilized for two positions.
One might be surprised that more people were not promoted from within. Common sense suggests otherwise. In
those departments where leadership changes were necessary, the previous leaders did not inspire their employees to
greatness, to say the least. Although there were some people
with potential, the departments where leadership replace-

ments were necessary just did not have the kind of talent that would have made internal promotion a good strategy. There were two exceptions, however—housekeeping and emergency room. A supervisor in housekeeping with a tremendous passion for learning and an excellent ability to motivate employees was promoted. Although she had only two months' experience in the hospital prior to her promotion, we decided to take a chance on her. She has responded by developing into an excellent executive housekeeper.

In our emergency room, a different internal promotion approach was utilized. There were no candidates for internal promotion in the emergency room itself. However, an operating room nurse was identified with excellent leadership skills and potential. It was an unconventional move, but she was promoted to emergency room department director. Initially, our emergency room physicians were against this move. They wanted someone with emergency room nursing experience. We stressed that leadership skills were more important than clinical skills for department director positions. They reluctantly agreed to give it a try. She too has developed into an excellent department director. Even the emergency room physicians are happy.

BUYING TIME

The necessity to recruit 11 new department directors brought with it the challenge of temporarily managing some departments. The time that director positions were vacant ranged from two weeks for internal promotions to 10 months for one of the particularly difficult recruitments, laboratory. The average time for department director positions remaining open was about four months. Positions could have been filled faster in almost all cases. But selection decisions were delayed until a candidate who met our high expectations was identified.

Departments were managed in the interim utilizing two approaches. Vice presidents served as ad hoc department directors in several instances. For six months the vice president of nursing filled in as the maternity department director in addition to her vice presidential duties. The vice president of professional services doubled as the director of education for several months while this recruitment was proceeding. This approach had several unexpected benefits. It gave the vice presidents a great deal of credibility because they were seen as willing to get into the ranks and help hold things together. It also motivated the vice presidents to keep the searches active since the longer the jobs were open, the longer they had to substitute as department directors.

Another interim approach which worked well was to utilize temporary assistance from outside the hospital. Through our affiliation with the University of Wisconsin Hospital and Clinics, two excellent *locum tenens* department directors were made available to the hospital for laboratory and dietary departments. This was beneficial to us since it held the departments together. It was also beneficial for University Hospital since it gave two of their first-line supervisors the experience of temporarily managing a department, which helped develop their management skills. Both interim management approaches enabled us to buy time and hold out for the very best permanent replacements.

The recruitment of 11 new department directors gave us a tremendous opportunity to put together a strong management team. The best of the old management group were retained and new strengths were added through recruitment and internal promotions. Although the recruitment period was challenging, the end results certainly justified the effort. Today, Beloit Memorial Hospital has one of the strongest management groups anywhere.

LESSONS OF HINDSIGHT

As hard as we tried, a perfect track record in recruiting was not achieved. Eleven new department directors and two new vice presidents were recruited. One big mistake was made. Even though there was an excellent interview and reference checking protocol in place, one individual was hired who did not meet our expectations. In hindsight, it was evident that the individual did not meet our expectations almost immediately after being hired. However, his vice president tried valiantly for about six months to bring the individual into line. I neglected to teach him what I learned the hard way 15 years previously.

New vice presidents sometimes get the idea that there is no department head that they cannot salvage and inspire to greatness if they try hard enough. Through experience they learn that some individuals just do not respond. One such individual was hired into our new team. Unfortunately the decision to replace him took too long. When a recruiting mistake is made, it is best to admit it, make the necessary changes and move on. No matter how hard they try, all executives make recruitment mistakes. What separates the winners from the also-rans is the ability to admit those mistakes and take the necessary action to correct the error—even if it means starting a recruitment all over again.

CHAPTER ELEVEN

A New Corporate Culture

HOW DOES A LEADER assimilate 13 new managers into an organization? Where does one start? Our approach was to create a "management culture" for department directors and vice presidents. That culture was then translated into an organizational culture for all employees. Culture is a nebulous term. In this context culture means a set of expectations and a framework for management to set good examples for others. Each organization has a unique culture. Sometimes an organization develops a culture in absentia, with little or no management intervention. The CEO should establish the organization's culture, for both management and employees. Creating a new culture was one of my personal priorities in year two.

LEADING BY EXAMPLE

The first step in establishing our management culture was to make some subtle changes in top management behavior. These changes were immediately observed by other members of the management staff. For example, soon after arriving in Beloit I discontinued the previous administration's practice of having department head meetings every other week which were 90 percent social and 10 percent business.

When I attended my first department head meeting I was appalled to find a collection of cakes, cookies and pies spread out all over the conference table. Department head meetings had been a place for having dessert and a little casual conversation rather than a place to conduct business. The girth of some of the department directors gave ample evidence of this approach's impact. Desserts were soon banished from the conference room and department head meetings were scheduled monthly. Their format was changed too. The meetings were used to communicate the status of the organization and the expectations I had for the managers.

The next example came in the area of work ethic. It was apparent almost immediately that the work ethic of the top management and middle management was more lax than I desired. It was not uncommon for vice presidents and department directors to be working six or seven hours a day and coming and going as they pleased. Coming in on the weekends or in evening or night hours to check on the operations of their departments was absolutely unheard of. That quickly changed. The dismissal of a vice president with particularly dismal work habits was the first move. The 12 hour a day work habits of myself and the other vice presidents quickly made it evident that hard work and constant checking of the operations during the off hours was expected. This led to some interesting discoveries.

Engineering staff members were sleeping on the job at night, nursing staff members were conducting love affairs on company time and various staff members were conducting personal business on hospital property on hospital time, to name a few. One of the worst examples of abuse was a member of the laboratory staff who ran a full-time real estate business from his work bench. To add insult to injury, he was a supervisor!

Personal integrity was another area that was quickly stressed. Under the previous administration, it was not uncommon for employees, department directors or even vice presidents to utilize hospital property for personal interest or gain. Vice presidents thought nothing of bringing their cars into the maintenance shop for repair work on hospital time or building trailers for their boats with hospital materials and hospital equipment. These practices quickly came to a halt. I let it be known throughout the hospital that it was no longer permissible to use hospital time or property for personal benefit.

Another area which got immediate attention was personal appearance of the management and their offices. Offices were cleaned up, and a dress code was informally implemented which confirmed that department directors were no longer welcome if they were tieless, wearing old, worn-out shoes or outfits suitable for bowling. I remember one department head who wore loud plaid sports coats with unmatched plaid pants and white patent leather shoes. The clown look went by the wayside rather quickly and more formal business attire became the rule of the day.

About half of the managers responded very well to these changes. The half that didn't either retired, were replaced or left the community to take other positions where white patent leather shoes and circus costumes were acceptable.

CREATING A NEW CULTURE

After articulating new management expectations, the next task was to identify the principles that really captured what the new leadership stood for. I labeled these principles "corporate values." They were first articulated to management and ultimately to all employees. Five corporate values were identified which defined the new corporate culture of Beloit Memorial Hospital: honesty and integrity; pride and quality; hard work; communication; and customer service.

How do you teach values to 700 employees? A little bit at a time. The job of articulating corporate values to our entire staff took a year. This was just the beginning. Once values were articulated, they had to be constantly reinforced if the leadership expected them to be practiced continually.

The vice presidents and I took on the formidable task of instilling our five corporate values into our work force. The approach used was similar to that of Jan Carlzon when he took over the troubled SAS Airlines in 1980. Carlzon and his top management group personally articulated their corporate values to all 20,000 SAS employees. After learning of Carlzon's impressive accomplishments, we decided to emulate him.

The process began at a series of special required attendance meetings for all employees. At those meetings, I articulated the five corporate values and what they meant to our organization.

I reinforced the need for having corporate values in the first place as a way to set our organization apart from our competition. The issue of job security was stressed in these meetings. I told the staff if we succeeded in practicing these corporate values that Beloit would surpass the competition and that everyone's job would be more secure in the future. The five corporate values were not original nor are they taught in the MBA curriculum at Harvard Business School. They are, however, the basis of what our leadership represents.

The four vice presidents and I each took one of the corporate values and developed a special employee presentation on that value. A five-part series of corporate value meetings was conducted throughout year two of the turnaround to articulate and reinforce our corporate values. Each of us utilized a slightly different approach to teach our assigned corporate value to employees. The special corporate value meetings were required attendance for all staff. It took a great deal of time and effort to prepare the value meetings. We went to considerable lengths to ensure that each employee got the message. In total, over 4,000 paid man-hours were invested in the corporate value meetings.

The honesty and integrity value was presented utilizing a well-known local judge. A special videotape was prepared covering interviews between the judge and staff members exchanging opinions about honesty and integrity. This was a particularly effective program. It covered a wide range of issues from patient confidentiality to cheating on sick time. The judge led the employees into defining honesty and integrity in a hospital context. He was excellent, and the video was well received by employees. The pride and quality value meetings were preceeded by an employee essay contest. All employees were invited to participate by writing a brief essay on what pride and quality meant to them. The winning essays were assembled into a book and distributed to all employees as part of the meeting for the pride and quality corporate value. The personal examples ranged from going the extra mile for a dying patient's family to making sure the garnishes on meal trays were perfect. Using the creativity of our employees helped define pride and quality in a very personal context.

The hard work value was illustrated by a homemade slide presentation. Slides stressed the importance of working together as a team. The communication value was illustrated by a video program which utilized employees and supervisors as the actors. Several 10-minute shows were put together which illustrated the best and the worst examples of communication, especially as it applied to patients. These programs were funny and extremely well put together.

The customer service value was illustrated through the use of a slide presentation which I put together. For about two weeks, I carried a camera with me in my rounds throughout the hospital and photographed various situations throughout the hospital which showed good examples and bad examples of customer service and attention to detail. This show was the last act in our series of corporate value meetings. We chose to home grow most of the corporate value material rather than to purchase videos and slide programs available from the outside. Much of the available material for employees is trendy "guest relations" hype. I was looking for something more permanent than smile training and slogans. In hindsight, I think our employees got the message more directly from our own programs.

During year two, the management team and I looked for opportunities to translate the five corporate values into everyday practice. For example, the process of reinforcing honesty and integrity was started by terminating people who stole from the hospital or who lied and got caught. Previously, management looked the other way when employees were stealing. When employees lied about things like sick time, more often than not management had ignored it. With the introduction of corporate values, employees began to be terminated for stealing and lying. This quickly became known throughout the organization.

Pride and quality standards were also reinforced. For example, employees who came to work looking like an unmade bed were sent home and told not to come back until they could present a professional appearance. Quality of work standards were also elevated. This was reinforced particularly in the nursing units, where patient care errors had never received much notice unless a patient was severely harmed. Even then, only minor discipline like a verbal warning was applied. Suspending and even terminating employees who made significant patient care errors was initiated. Hard work standards were also reinforced for the first time in the hospital. Employees discovered sleeping were terminated instead of being given a slap on the wrist and told to drink more coffee. Also terminated were several supervisors who had been cheating the hospital for years by getting paid for a full day's work when their department directors and even the administration knew they were only working part-time.

The communication value was reinforced by practicing what we preached. Quarterly assembly meetings, monthly departmental meetings and a new employee representative position to reinforce the communication value throughout the organization were created. The customer service value was reinforced by providing a positive example for the staff. When customers were dissatisfied, the vice presidents made it a point to personally follow up. Vice presidents even made visits to patients' homes after discharge to personally hear their complaints and either resolve the complaint or provide an apology. For example, the vice president of professional services visited the home of a radiology patient who developed a severe bruise at the injection site for contrast media for a CT scan. The vice president extended his apology for the patient's discomfort and invited her to return to the emergency room later in the day to have the bruise examined by the emergency room physician at no charge. After several months of seeing the management practice customer service on a personal level, employees got the message and jumped on the bandwagon.

Once the values were articulated through the year-long series of special meetings, constant reinforcement was necessary. Three reinforcement approaches were used. For all new employees, I present a 30-minute synopsis of our corporate values in new employee orientation. Next, in quarterly assembly meetings I always pick one of the values for a 10-minute refresher. Lastly, our department directors and vice presidents constantly reinforce the corporate values in their day-to-day interchange with employees.

TEACHING THE TEACHERS

Articulation of the corporate values was for the most part done by the vice presidents and myself. As new department directors came on board, my attention turned to developing the middle and upper management staff to fit the organization's new expectations and culture. Some hospitals assign management development to a person or department. My approach was to accept management development as part of the CEOs' and vice presidents' ongoing responsibilities. The vice presidents and I made a commitment to be the management teachers rather than relying on a development department or the use of outside teaching consultants. I'm convinced that this produces much longer lasting results.

The task of management development was initiated by creating the "Spring Lecture Series" in year two. The lecture series took the form of presenting five core management subjects to the vice presidents and department directors.

These core subjects were taught by myself and the vice presidents. The subjects were:

The Role of Management

Effective Communication

Motivating and Evaluating Employees

Managing Perceptions and Attitudes

The Role of Marketing

The Role of Management class gave me an opportunity to reinforce new management position descriptions and articulate how managers themselves were to be evaluated and rewarded for success. Lecture material and case presentations were used to illustrate key points. The classes on communication focused on communicating with superiors, peers and employees. Again, practical case presentations were used to illustrate the key points. The motivation and evaluation program stressed praise and discipline as equally effective methods for achieving desired employee results. The perceptions and attitudes classes stressed the everyday situations with which all managers are confronted. The Role of Marketing class stressed that marketing, as I defined it, was 10 percent advertising and 90 percent creation of a service attitude among employees for the everyday contacts between employees and customers.

Each of these subjects required two to three hours of classroom and discussion time. The core presentations were videotaped for future use with new managers. When the department directors and vice presidents got used to the approach, it gave us a sense of camaraderie and joint learning that simply would not have been possible if we merely hired outside teachers to do the work for us.

To supplement the classroom approach, a bi-annual management retreat was created for department directors and vice presidents. These retreats were half business and half pleasure. Retreat days began with a half day learning session followed by lunch and a half day of recreation.

These retreats generally utilized a recently published management book to stimulate discussion. For instance, *A Passion For Excellence, Service America* and *In Search of Excellence* were used. Retreats usually took the form of approximately an hour of presentation by myself and the vice presidents, followed by group discussions by the department directors. Group discussions centered around extracting ideas from the books being reviewed and applying them to the hospital business in general and our hospital specifically. Many of the creative customer relations approaches now practiced by our hospital originated in these management retreat sessions.

MANAGEMENT DEVELOPMENT IS NEVER FINISHED

Although a considerable amount of time and effort was spent articulating corporate values and developing our management staff, it is an ongoing process. Monthly department director meetings are used to reinforce the corporate values and management expectations. The spring lecture series is repeated every year using two different tracks. First, the core sessions are repeated for all of the new department directors who have been hired during the previous year. Second, three or four new sessions are introduced each year which meet the specific needs of the hospital in that year. Also, new books and films are constantly being selected to illustrate and reinforce corporate values. The *In Search of Excellence* and *A Passion For Excellence* videotapes were particularly helpful in this regard. All this management development takes a great deal of time and effort, but it was worth it. It was vital to our turnaround and even more important in our future success.

LESSONS OF HINDSIGHT

It took awhile, but it did finally dawn on us that in all of our efforts to upgrade hospital employees and management, one key group was omitted. This hit home one day about six months after the employee corporate value presentations were completed when I stopped a nurse in the hallway and chewed her out. She was in a poorly pressed uniform and had a surly and uncommunicative attitude. She stood out like a sore thumb. As I raised my voice and prepared to suspend her on the spot, she raised her hand defensively and said, "Hey, don't pick on me, I work for the clinic."

As it turned out, she worked for the community's large clinic across the street. She was in the hospital only to deliver some materials to a physician. In all of our efforts to upgrade hospital employees, it became evident to our patients and the community that some of the employees and managers who worked for physician groups were not in tune with the new approaches and attitudes of the hospital staff. If we had it to do all over again, the physicians' office staffs and managers would have been invited to be part of the hospital's corporate value training programs from the beginning. In that way, all staff could have learned together and presented a more uniformly positive attitude to the customers which we both served.

CHAPTER TWELVE

Listen to the Customers

*A*S THE PROCESS of articulating
corporate values got underway, the hospital was faced with
the difficult decision of how to differentiate itself from the
competition. Marketers call this "positioning." Market research confirmed that our community and patients felt that
the hospital was not listening to them. Listening and responding to customer needs was selected as our positioning
strategy. Adding 200 beds, doubling the medical staff or doing open heart surgery were out of the question. But our research showed that our competitors were still listening to
themselves, not their customers. So the opportunity to be
the best listeners was seized as our competitive edge.

GO RIGHT TO THE TOP

I felt that it was imperative to have our new listening strategies emanate from the top. Taking a cue from hotel managers, a president's welcome card was created for our
patients. The idea was to give a welcome card to each inpatient the day of admission. A sample of this card is shown in
figure 5. Each day, my secretary begins her morning by feed-
ing the admitting list from the previous 24 hours into our
word processing unit. The word processor then types

FIGURE 5

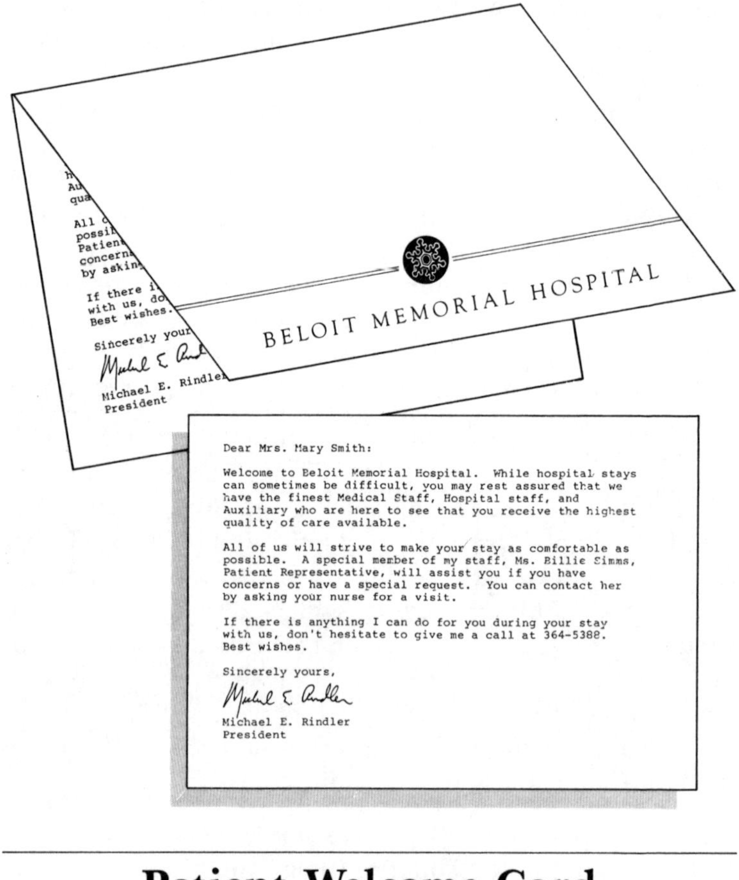

Dear Mrs. Mary Smith:

Welcome to Beloit Memorial Hospital. While hospital stays can sometimes be difficult, you may rest assured that we have the finest Medical Staff, Hospital staff, and Auxiliary who are here to see that you receive the highest quality of care available.

All of us will strive to make your stay as comfortable as possible. A special member of my staff, Ms. Billie Simms, Patient Representative, will assist you if you have concerns or have a special request. You can contact her by asking your nurse for a visit.

If there is anything I can do for you during your stay with us, don't hesitate to give me a call at 364-5388. Best wishes.

Sincerely yours,

Michael E. Rindler

Michael E. Rindler
President

BELOIT MEMORIAL HOSPITAL

Patient Welcome Card

newly admitted patient names on each greeting card. When I arrive for work my first task is to sign each greeting card and add a handwritten postscript if I happen to know the patient personally. We average 20 admissions per day, so the whole operation takes about ten minutes of secretarial time and about five minutes of my own time daily.

One important feature of this program is the way the cards are delivered. My secretary delivers each card personally and welcomes patients to the hospital on my behalf. An unexpected benefit of this personal delivery is that my secretary often brings back useful information about the attitude of patients and sometimes identifies little problems before they become big ones. Occasionally I deliver the cards, or have one of the vice presidents do it to reinforce the interest of top management in our patients. For example, one newly admitted patient said she was very pleased with the care, but that because her bedside telephone had two different numbers, she was unsure of which one to give her family members and friends. A quick call to the engineering department cleared up this small but important problem immediately.

The unique feature of this welcome card is a special phone number. It gives our patients direct access to the president without going through any middle managers or secretaries. I answer this phone personally at all times when I am in my office. When I am away from the phone, my secretary answers, and I return the call immediately when I return. At the time this welcome card was implemented, it was the first of its kind in the country. It may still be the only one. When customers know that the chief executive officer is willing to listen to their compliments and complaints, it makes a positive impression on them and a powerful statement to the rest of the organization about responsiveness.

WHERE ARE MY RICE KRISPIES?

I worried, prior to implementing this system, that my day would be spent tied to the telephone. Experience has shown

that concern was unwarranted. I receive about 10 calls during an average week. About half of these calls are compliments about a physician or staff member who has done a
particularly nice job, and the patient wants me to know
about it. These calls provide an opportunity to send the staff
member a thank you note for his or her excellent work.

The other half of the calls are negative. I have found
that when patients feel strongly enough to call me they are
generally extremely upset and want immediate attention.
No matter how bad the call is, however, the direct phone
line gives me an opportunity to turn negative stories
into positive ones. I recall receiving a phone call one afternoon from a very upset patient who had been discharged
about a month previously. She had been told several weeks
previously by our business office that she would be issued a
refund check due to a charging error. She waited for the
$200 to arrive, but it never did. After several attempts to se-
cure the refund by going through channels she gave up and
called me. The woman was of limited means and really
needed the refund which was due her. When I received her
angry call, I apologized profusely and promised to resolve
the matter that day. I then went across the hall to the business office, had her check prepared immediately, and drove
to the woman's home to deliver it with my personal apolo-
gies. When I got back to the hospital I had a few stern words
for the business office about its poor response to this woman's plight.

Several months after this incident, our market research
firm was conducting a focus group among community residents. One of the good stories presented was the delivery of
that refund check by the hospital's CEO. The story was
fourth hand by the time it got to the focus group, but the
fact that it showed up at all left me with a lasting impression
that personal and prompt attention can turn a negative experience into a positive one.

I recall another serious complaint from a young mother
who had delivered her first baby in our facility several
months previously. She called and complained about the en-

tire range of her hospital experience, from the attitude of our nursing staff to the cleanliness of our rooms. Since maternity was one of our better services, I was extremely concerned. In this case, I turned the complaint over to the vice presidents of support services and nursing for personal follow up. They visited the new mother in her home to discuss her complaints. After learning firsthand how upset she was about her care, they returned several days later with flowers as a gesture of apology. We later learned that this woman's negative experience had been totally overpowered by the fact that two vice presidents visited her home and personally apologized for her bad hospital experience.

One more illustration. I got a call one morning about 9 a.m. from an extremely agitated patient. She had been in the hospital one week and had no nearby friends or relatives. She informed me that she had been eating Rice Krispies for breakfast for the last 25 years. In spite of her requests for Rice Krispies she had received substitutes every day of her seven-day hospitalization. She denigrated her entire hospital experience simply because she couldn't get Rice Krispies for breakfast. A quick phone call to the director of dietary yielded the embarrassing information that we were out of Rice Krispies. I dispatched the red-faced director of dietary across the street to the grocery store to buy a box of Rice Krispies, which was promptly delivered to my office. I then took five minutes to visit the patient and present her with her personal box of Rice Krispies. She was overwhelmed by this small gesture. Instead of complaining for the rest of her two-week stay about the unresponsiveness of the dietary department, she told her friends and neighbors about the hospital president's gift of her personal box of Rice Krispies.

The dietary director's attitude about the incident was interesting. She was angry and pointed out that she felt demeaned to be sent on a shopping trip for a patient. Her attitude was that the patient should have adjusted to corn flakes. The dietary director now practices her profession at another facility. There are countless stories like these in which negative experiences have been turned into positive ones by quick response and easy access to top management. This approach can be a tremendously powerful marketing strategy for any hospital.

THE LEE IACOCCA ADS

Another symbol which confirmed our commitment to listening was the design of our newspaper advertising campaign. Although the campaign will be discussed in more detail in chapter 15, a copy of one of the ads is illustrated in figure 6. This ad campaign carried the same special phone number as the patient greeting cards. It literally invited citizens to call if they had suggestions and ideas for improvement. During the past several years, I have received many excellent ideas over this phone line. For example, the front entrance doors were made easier to open for wheelchair patients after I received a suggestion from a handicapped patient. A "treat first ask questions later" program was implemented in our emergency room after an irate patient called and accused us of being more interested in paperwork than patient care. A "courtesy discharge" program was installed in our cashier's office which emulated fast checkout procedures in fine hotels. The new system eliminated the paperwork associated with checking out of the hospital. A wealth of good ideas are out there if the hospital takes the time to listen to its customers.

Another listening commitment was implemented using a patient representative program with a unique twist. Many hospitals have patient representative programs. However, our approach of giving the patient representative a checkbook and the authority to use it is unique. Many times patient representatives merely listen to patient problems and pass them along to someone else to resolve. Our patient representative does some of this. However, she also carries a checkbook with my authority to use it when an immediate remedy is possible. If someone's contact lenses are lost by the staff, she writes out a check to replace them on the spot.

FIGURE 6

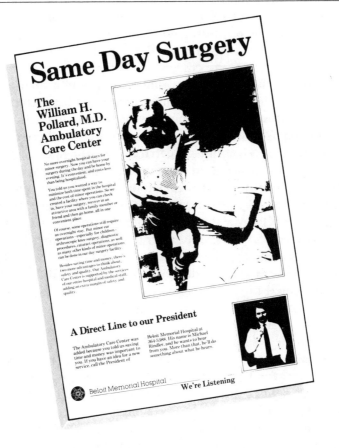

We're Listening Campaign

If an item of clothing is lost or dentures are damaged when being removed, a check is issued to replace them on the spot. In the course of one year, about $2,000 are spent on these immediate response items. The goodwill generated by the immediate responses is worth far more than the cash expenses. Sometimes the checks worked marketing miracles.

One such check was written for $10 for "dog sitting." An elderly gentleman had been admitted in late afternoon and needed someone to watch his dogs for the night. The gentleman had suffered a heart attack and had no friends or relatives living with him. The patient representative solved the problem by having his dog taken to a boarding kennel. The $10 spent having his dogs taken care of that evening was worth $1,000 of advertising. The patient told everyone who would listen for the next year about how responsive Beloit Memorial Hospital was to his special needs. The patient representative checkbook is a great example of how a few dollars can be multiplied a hundred times in their marketing impact.

A VICE PRESIDENTIAL RECEPTIONIST

Every one of our vice presidents created their own special techniques for listening to their division's customers. The vice president of finance began randomly calling several patients each week to determine whether or not they could understand their bills. These phone calls were one of the reasons our billing nomenclature was completely redone so that individuals without a Ph.D. in computer science or medicine could read and understand them. He also makes a point of calling a few patients every week to determine their experiences in the admitting and cashier's office, both of which are under his responsibility.

Our vice president of support services makes a point of personally passing several patient meal trays each week and then interviewing patients about how good or bad the food is. He also interviews a number of employee customers every week. For example, he speaks with members of the nursing staff about the quality and availability of supplies and linen. He also checks directly with staff members to find out how well the equipment they work with is maintained by the engineering department. Our vice president of professional services makes it a point to call several patients each week who have utilized lab and x-ray services. He also spends a few minutes every week in our lobby manning the reception desk and assisting patients being discharged into their car. Our vice president of nursing makes it a point to spend enough time on the nursing stations every week to answer several patient lights and deliver pain medications when ordered. She too randomly calls patients at home to determine their experience with nursing services, and she checks constantly with our physicians to verify that the nursing staff is on its toes.

DEPARTMENT DIRECTORS LISTEN TOO

Department directors began to notice my own listening activities and those of the vice presidents and created some unique ones of their own. Listening and staying close to customers is now part of the fabric of our organization. Our customers know they can contact anyone in management, from myself to the vice presidents to the department heads, and expect a prompt response.

Our laboratory director routinely contacts patients to determine how well phlebotomists are doing. Our radiology director calls patients to verify that pre-exam preparation instructions and scheduling is working satisfactorily. Our dietary director personally conducts patient interviews to determine satisfaction with the food. Our intensive care unit nursing director calls patients several weeks after discharge to determine how well her nursing staff did in dealing with families. Our operating room director makes post-surgery visits and phone calls to patients. She also sees that her staff calls every single outpatient on the day following surgery to verify that their experience was satisfactory and that they have no residual questions.

Our emergency room director calls some patients personally and has set up a system so that every patient is contacted a day or two following their ER visit. Another adaptation of this approach is the patient interviews conducted by the director of human resources. She visits several patients every week to check perceptions on employee attitudes and skill levels. She understands that ultimately she is responsible for hiring excellent people. Who better to check with than the patients themselves to determine whether or not she is achieving that goal?

All of our department directors listen to their customers. Their approaches are ongoing and creative. Their success was evident when follow up market research studies became available. More on that later.

EMPLOYEES LISTEN TOO

Last, and certainly not least, employees and physicians began getting into listening in year two. One particularly good example was the creation of a vascular team for our peripheral vascular surgery patients. Under the direction of our vascular surgeon, a multi-disciplinary team of nurses, physicians, operating room technicians and radiology personnel was assembled for the purpose of improving communication and quality for their patients. They began their task by creating pre-surgical visits for patients and family members to fully explain the surgical procedures.

These were not your typical "in and out" consent signing visits. They were high quality visits with plenty of time for all parties to ask questions and have them answered. The vascular team then implemented follow up contacts with family members during the actual operation. Most vascular surgery procedures are lengthy, and the surgeon now routinely dispatches a member of the surgery team to communicate with family members during the procedure to let them know how the operation is proceeding. Following the case, the team makes post-surgical visits to answer questions for the patients and family members. A special discharge information packet was assembled by the physician and nurses for patients to refer to when they have left the hospital. They added one last touch, a business card, with the team's phone numbers so that any patient could reach a member of the team at any time following surgery if there were a question or concern. This example of multidisciplinary teamwork really confirmed that our employees and physicians had gotten the listening message.

Knowing that employees were responding, one last step was taken to facilitate listening. Each employee in the hospital received a set of business cards for personal use. The business cards contain information about the employees which does not fit easily on a name tag. For example, a laboratory technician might want the credentials "BS, MT, ASCP" on their name tag. Although space might not permit all credentials to be placed on the name tag, they can certainly be printed on a personal business card.

Every employee was given the opportunity to spell out what they wanted on their business cards, including titles, credentials and even a brief comment. Then the business cards were printed and distributed to employees with the request that they use them when interacting with patients or family members. Beloit Memorial Hospital may be the only hospital in the country which gives every employee a set of business cards and encourages their use.

One might think employees would be reluctant to use business cards. Nothing could be further from the truth. I learned that on the day they were distributed during an assembly meeting. Following the question and answer period the business cards were distributed and I was immediately cornered by an ICU nurse. She wanted to remind me of the going away party for a retiring nurse the following week. She asked me if I would contribute two dollars to her going away dinner. I readily agreed. To be sure I wouldn't forget, she peeled off one of her newly printed business cards and wrote on the back, "You owe me two dollars." Later that evening as I was undressing, the business card fell out of my pocket. My wife was quite curious about why I had a woman's business card in my pocket with a notation on the back that I owed her money.

In practice, the business cards are used constantly by employees. CT technicians routinely pass out the cards to let patients and family members know they can call back at any time with questions about their procedures. Nurses use the cards with discharged patients to let them know they can call at any time with questions about their care. Housekeepers use the cards to let patients know whom to call in the event that they need more towels or a change of bed linen. Engineering employees use them when they fix items like shower heads in patient rooms, so that patients will know whom to call if the fix did not resolve the problem. I have been pleasantly surprised by the creativity of our staff in using their cards. The small cost of printing them is far outweighed by the tremendous sense of pride that employees have in carrying the cards and the creativity that they demonstrate by using them.

LESSONS OF HINDSIGHT

On the positive side, our experience confirmed that an organization of seven hundred employees can be sensitized to listening. This formidable task was accomplished in a year. But it takes a tremendous amount of reinforcement to maintain a high level of listening. Our success enabled us to create a meaningful advertising campaign with the simple theme, "We're Listening."

On the negative side, it was learned that once an expectation is created in the community, it can never be relaxed. Now, when a complaint is not resolved with lightning speed, customers think we have stopped listening and caring. We are hostage to our own success. It could be worse.

CHAPTER THIRTEEN

Marketing and Community Relations

BELOIT MEMORIAL HOSPITAL re-
sisted the temptation to advertise heavily during the early
stages of the turnaround. It was decided to work first on the
substance of patient relations and patient care quality and
leave advertising and community relations until later. The
timing of our first advertising efforts was considered critical. If it came too soon, the hospital would not have enough
credibility in the community for advertising to work. On
the other hand, if it came too late, advertising efforts of
competitors would continue eroding our patient base.

The first major advertising campaign came in year two,
after completion of strategic slate goals. The assertion that
good marketing and community relations are 10 percent advertising and 90 percent paying attention to the things that
matter for our patients was our philosophy. The essence of
marketing in the healthcare setting is producing satisfied
customers who will tell their friends and neighbors about
their positive experiences. Our marketing and community
relations strategies were co-mingled to the point where it
was not really clear where community relations left off and
marketing began. That is just the way we wanted it. It is important to note that I do not believe in marketers per se. We

had no vice president of marketing. The vice presidents, department directors and I were collectively the marketers for Beloit Memorial Hospital.

OUR FIRST COMMUNITY RELATIONS COUP

The vanguard of our community relations program was to take advantage of opportunities to publicize the positive aspects of the hospital's progress. The first such opportunity came early in year two with the fifteenth anniversary of the hospital's opening. This milestone was seized as an opportunity to promote the many positive changes which had taken place in the hospital.

The first break came when the governor of Wisconsin agreed to attend our fifteenth anniversary events. The persistent efforts of our director of community relations were responsible for this success. Once the governor was committed, a two-day open house was planned which combined hospital tours for community residents, positive news coverage, free health screening and a series of press conferences.

The fifteenth anniversary open house was our first major teamwork success. Physicians, volunteers, management and employees all worked together for several months to prepare for the open house events. When the weekend of the open house finally arrived, the hospital looked wonderful and the positive news coverage was gratifying. Over two thousand people from the community took advantage of free screening tests and tours of the hospital. This turned out to be the most successful community relations event ever undertaken by the hospital. The positive newspaper articles and subsequent letters to the editor continued for weeks afterwards. Later that year Beloit Memorial Hospital's fifteenth anniversary open house won the Wisconsin Public Relations Society's most prestigious award for hospitals.

HITTING THE SPEAKING TRAIL

Another successful community relations strategy was the availability of myself and members of the management and medical staff to give community presentations about the hospital. An extensive slide program was prepared which covered the hospital's market research findings and our commitment to resolving the identified problems. The slide program also highlighted the new facilities built, equipment bought and physicians recruited to provide better quality care. These speaking engagements were highly successful. They ranged from groups of 150 or so at the local Rotary to groups as small as 10 community residents in Sunday morning church groups. In total, members of the medical staff and management staff gave over 50 community presentations during the second year of our turnaround. These face-to-face presentations helped the community understand how hard the hospital was trying to improve itself. It also gave community residents an opportunity to ask questions about rumors. These exchanges gave us the chance to turn negatives into positives.

For example, the staff reductions gained a great deal of negative press in the local newspaper. Cost cutting, especially when it includes staff reductions, has a generally bad connotation in healthcare. The subject of cost cutting came up frequently during community presentations. It gave us an opportunity to talk about the many common sense cost cutting measures mentioned earlier. Presentations enabled us to show how the quality of care at the hospital had been improved rather than diminished by cost cutting. It also gave us an opportunity to talk about management staff reductions in a positive light. The community reacted favorably when we explained that the reduction in management salaries enabled us to put more money back into improving the equipment and services of the hospital. Although the speaking circuit can be strenuous, the effort was well worth it.

A variation of the speaking engagement approach em-

ployed during our second year was community leader briefings. Approximately 30 individuals were brought into the
hospital for extensive briefing and tours. There were two
types of community leaders that we were interested in
reaching. The obvious leaders were those who led the major corporations, held key political posts and ran prominent
service organizations.

The second type of leaders were opinion leaders. These
were major car dealers, real estate brokers, ministers and re-
tailers. We met with both types of community leaders on
several occasions and gave extensive presentations on the
hospital's prior problems, efforts to resolve those problems
and our plans for the future. By reaching the community
leaders in a very direct personal fashion, we turned most
doubters into strong hospital supporters.

BACK IN THE NEWSPAPER AGAIN

The hospital avoided the local newspaper like the plague
during the first year of the turnaround. Since most of the activities were negative, such as layoffs and management firings, I felt it best to say as little as possible. During the
second year the approach softened. Access to the hospital
by newspaper reporters was improved and news releases began to flow again. Courting reporters and editors also began.
Although our efforts were not well received at first, eventually the newspaper forgave us for our early reluctance to be
open and began giving us excellent and balanced coverage.
Our director of community relations developed a close relationship with the editorial and reporting staff at the local
newspaper. This relationship facilitated the paper's need for
timely news and our interest in receiving positive media exposure.

At the same time, members of the medical staff and
management staff were encouraged to go on local TV and
talk shows. Radio talk shows were particularly effective in
getting the message out to the community about new and
improved hospital services.

BABY PICNICS AND CHRISTMAS TREES

Another community relations approach started in year two was opening the hospital to community groups. Meeting rooms such as the board room and auditorium were made available for local community agencies for their own meetings. This gave access to community groups that sorely needed professional meeting space. Renting unused office space at the hospital to health-related community agencies was also started. For example, the local hospice group rented space which helped meet expectations for professional office space while reducing travel time for hospice volunteers to and from the hospital.

The Auxiliary also created some excellent new programs which gave the hospital excellent visibility in the community. Two good examples were "Baby Alumni" picnics and the "Love Light Christmas Tree" program. The Baby Alumni picnic was an excellent promotion effort for our maternity service. It involved a day-long series of events during the summer in which all the babies who were born in our hospital during the previous five years and their families were invited to a lawn party. The day's events included children's carnival rides, birthday cake and cookies, games and puppet shows, free balloons and much more. The event is now conducted annually and draws about one thousand children and their families. It's a wonderful thing seeing parents coming back to the hospital to talk to the physicians and nurses who delivered their newborns. The social interaction and the great time had by all were great marketing for our maternity service.

The Auxiliary's Love Light Christmas Tree program was another innovation which created a great deal of positive press coverage for the hospital, and raised some money as well. Community residents could purchase a Christmas tree light for a loved one who had passed away or in honor of someone they wished to recognize. A special tree was planted in the hospital entrance to serve as the Love Light Tree. The lights cost only two dollars each, so individuals from all walks of life in the community were able to purchase one. Thousands of community residents purchased tree lights. Many of them attended the tree lighting ceremony which now takes place every year the week before Christmas. The local newspaper helped by printing the names of individuals who were being honored or remembered. They also gave the hospital several positive stories, including wonderful pictures of the tree lighting ceremony. Without question, the Auxiliary's new programs assisted greatly in opening up the hospital to the community.

ADVERTISING: OUR FIRST ATTEMPT

Our first major advertising campaign took place during the middle of year two. The urge to advertise before that time was resisted because the problems that the community had identified were not yet resolved. After achieving success on strategic slate items, it was time to let the community know the results. Market research provided the theme for the advertising campaign.

Initial market research confirmed that the community did not feel the hospital was responding to their needs. Residents in turn began leaving the community to seek healthcare services elsewhere. The responsiveness issue gave us the idea for the ad campaign theme. Since we had worked so hard on the strategic slate issues and since the issues themselves came from the community market research, it was decided to use a campaign theme of "We're Listening."

Initially, an advertising firm was hired to develop the campaign theme and ad design. It quickly became apparent that the working relationship between the hospital and advertising firm was not going to work out. From our point of view, it did not appear that they were responding to our needs. From their point of view, they thought we were a difficult, if not impossible, client. After several stormy meetings, we decided to complete the campaign on our own. Our ability to do this was enhanced considerably by the presence of talented people on the hospital staff. We were fortunate to have excellent writers, as well as photography and graphic design skills inhouse. A nearby, excellent printing firm was able to service our typesetting needs at a high level of quality and reasonable cost. The design theme chosen for the print campaign was a large photograph with approximately three hundred words of text to go with it. Each strategic slate problem was to have its own advertisement. Each advertisement also carried a unique tagline which included a small photograph of myself and an invitation to use my special, direct phone number for new ideas and questions about the hospital. Because of this tagline, it became locally known as "Michael Rindler's Lee Iacocca ad campaign."

The print campaign consisted of six separate advertisements. The first ad introduced the campaign by referring to the community market research and problems identified. Subsequent ads addressed five strategic slate issues: emergency medicine, patient convenience, high tech, physician specialists and responsiveness and attention to detail. Copies of the introductory ad and the High Tech ad are included as samples in figure 7.

Before launching the ad campaign, I previewed it to our physicians, employees and the board. Previewing the ads and making large blowups of the ads for the hospital lobby and cafeteria a month before the ad campaign actually began running worked well to thoroughly familiarize all hospital groups with the purpose and theme of the ad campaign. This helped our staff address questions from the community about why we were advertising. Since this was our first attempt at advertising, we wanted to be sure that employees knew that the amount of money invested was small compared with other patient service investments.

The response from the media and community toward our advertising campaign was gratifying. Since the ads featured "real people," the community quickly identified with the individuals and message. The community also responded well to the approach of admitting that the hospital

FIGURE 7

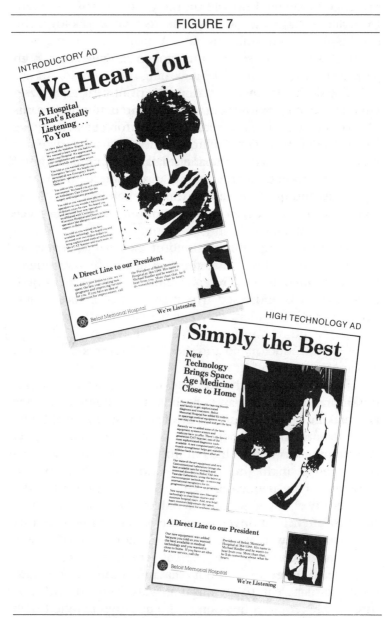

We're Listening Campaign

had some problems and was working hard to resolve them. Each of the six ads ran weekly for four weeks. In total, the campaign lasted six months. I received approximately five to ten calls per week from people in the community upon seeing the invitation to use my special phone number. Many superb ideas for improvement throughout the hospital came from these phone calls. For example, parking spaces available for senior citizens were expanded and the cafeteria schedule was changed to accommodate visitors and patients' families, to name just a few. The elimination of smoking in all patient rooms and creating a more home-like appearance for family lounges also came as a result of community phone calls to the president. The ad campaign and direct phone line to the president gave the community an opportunity to participate in improving the hospital. For the first time, the community had access to someone who would listen to their suggestions and act on them.

MORE ADVERTISING: GOOD NEWS AND BAD NEWS

Toward the end of year two, another series of ads were developed. The same design theme, with large photographs, small amount of text and a second small photograph and tagline was used. These ads highlighted our maternity service, physical medicine, surgery and nursing care. The ad design was essentially a testimonial. This ad series also was well-received in the community. Examples of these "real people" ads are pictured in figure 8.

One bad advertising experience did occur. Maternity service was our strongest service in terms of community perception. It was decided to do a major maternity campaign late in year two. I decided to try our luck again with an advertising agency. The ads were prepared utilizing a substantially different design layout than earlier campaigns. The ads were well written and elegantly designed. We thought that the campaign would be a big success.

FIGURE 8

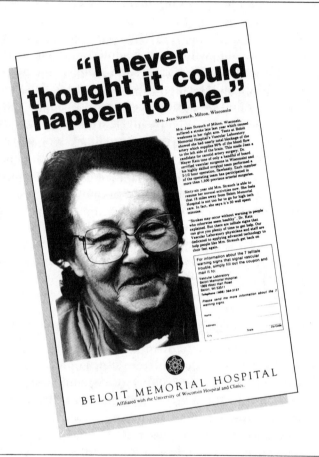

Testimonial Ad Sample

Wrong. More money was spent on that maternity campaign than on all our previous advertising efforts combined. For all of the money spent, the campaign had the worst response rate of any we had run. The ad photographs featured professional models, which was resented by some members of our community who notice such things. The response rate was so low that we concluded once and for all that hiring a good agency does not necessarily produce positive results. Although the advertising gurus say that clients should absolutely leave the professionals to their work, our experience proved just the contrary. Whenever the job was turned over to a professional ad firm, more money got spent for less positive results than when campaigns were produced locally.

In year two, some event-related advertising was also sponsored. For example, for the first time in several years, annual reports were published, which included summaries of new services and our financial and activity statistics. Our financial picture had been so bleak in recent years that public reports had ceased to be published. Now that there was something to be proud of, annual reports were again a positive source of advertising. Advertising during National Hospital Week, ads in special newspaper supplements on healthcare issues, ads for events like the annual awards for employees and so forth were used. Several years and thousands of dollars later, our conclusion is that these types of advertisements did little if anything for our image or business. They have since been discontinued.

Finally, billboards, shopping mall displays and other difficult-to-evaluate advertising strategies were initiated in year two. Also tried were county fair participation, display booths and the purchase of senior citizen walking trails in shopping malls to put our name before the public. It is difficult, if not impossible, to evaluate the effectiveness of these advertising efforts. Although they increase the hospital's visibility in the community, it is unclear whether they produced any positive results in terms of maintaining or increasing business. Hopefully, someone will invent an evaluation methodology which will enable hospitals to analyze costs and benefits of advertising better than we are able to today.

LESSONS OF HINDSIGHT

Although I avoided mentioning it earlier, one set of advertisements was produced during the first year of our turnaround. These advertisements were intended more to improve employee morale than to produce definite results. During the hospital's declining years, competing hospitals had begun advertising heavily in the local newspaper. Employees became more and more discouraged as the hospital's business declined and the visibility of other hospitals increased. To create an advertising presence about six months after the turnaround began, a series of maternity ads was produced.

Although the ads did accomplish getting our name in the newspaper, they did not accomplish much else. They were thrown together quickly with little physician input. They managed to offend the very group we were trying to promote. The ads were supposed to promote maternity services, which included both family practitioners and obstetricians. The family practitioner group had several weak physicians in terms of maternity capabilities. This was in stark contrast to the local obstetricians, who were extremely well thought of in the medical community and the patient community. With this dilemma in mind, the ads were structured to favor the obstetricians over the family practitioners. The ads even featured the obstetrician's office numbers and ignored the family practitioners. I made all the wrong decisions.

The family practitioners were furious. They felt ignored and insulted by the ads. They were not bashful about letting their feelings be known in the community and to hospital board members. The result was that I created a fire storm of bad feelings for no good reason.

Looking back on the experience, it was a mistake to

rush into publishing those ads in the first place. Beyond that, it was a mistake not to review more carefully the ad content with all the physicians who would be affected by it. Having done so would have probably eliminated the use of the obstetricians' phone numbers, the issue that created the most hard feelings. A valuable lesson was learned with this fiasco. Although it is important to retain control of the advertising process, it is equally important to involve physicians enough so that major mistakes and hard feelings can be avoided. It wasn't a fatal disaster, but it sure did hurt.

CHAPTER FOURTEEN

Achieving Results

BUILDING A NEW MANAGEMENT team, creating a corporate culture and implementing the hospital's first marketing efforts were directed at the strategic slate goal to improve responsiveness to customers. The vice presidents and I, in conjunction with the medical staff, produced successes in year two on each of the other five strategic slate goals. No magic was involved. Hard work, persistence and a fundamental belief that success was achievable inspired us. Fear of failure and subsequent loss of employment inspired us too.

THE LAST LAUGH WAS OURS

The old saying "He who laughs last laughs best" became the theme for recruitment of a new group of emergency medicine physicians. Beloit Memorial Hospital had been served by an outside contractor for emergency medicine physicians for about ten years. This arrangement had not worked satisfactorily, especially in the years immediately preceding the turnaround. The recruitment of a new group of emergency medicine physicians became our first strategic slate priority.

Our sights were set high. The goal became to settle for

nothing less than a new group of emergency medicine residency trained specialists. The group was to be locally based. This was especially important to our community image, which had been damaged by the "carpetbagger" perception of the contract physician group. The contract physicians chose to live in Madison, Milwaukee or Chicago. They never became part of the Beloit community.

The first move was to announce to our contract group that their services would be terminated nine months hence. They responded with a chuckle. They said our goal was unrealistic, unachievable. But the last laugh was to be ours. The recruitment started with assembling a search committee of management and physicians, headed by the vice president of professional services. The search committee used a multifaceted approach which included a physician search firm, journal advertisements, residency contacts and a direct mail campaign to residents in emergency medicine.

It was also decided to go public with the recruitment plans so that the community would know that the hospital was seeking a new group of emergency medicine physicians. Newspaper releases and our annual report announced our intentions. At first thought it might seem inappropriate to announce our intentions so publicly. But we wanted the community to know that relief was coming on the hospital problem which gave them the most concern. It never crossed our minds that we might fail and be subsequently embarrassed. The decision to go public was fortunate and ultimately gave us the recruitment break that brought success.

A physician search firm was hired to focus on the chief of emergency medicine position. The other recruitment strategies identified candidates for the three staff physician positions. It took five months of intensive efforts before any qualified candidates were identified. After interviewing ten physicians, the first round of candidates was exhausted without any chief or staff physicians that met our expectations. Then our big break arrived. The hospital's annual report in year two included a paragraph about the emergency medicine recruitment. The annual report was received by a physician in a nearby community who sent it to his son who was completing an emergency medicine residency in Akron, Ohio. This young physician was part of a group of four graduating residents who wanted to set up an emergency medicine practice in a midwest community.

After several weeks of telephone discussions and letter exchanges, the prospective physicians visited Beloit. The search committee was delighted with their credentials and their interest in our community. After a month of negotiations, it became apparent that the group was going to locate in one of two communities, and Beloit was still in the running. Serious negotiations followed with the group, and contract drafts were prepared. As the end of the negotiations neared, it became a horse race between our hospital and a nearby tertiary hospital. A dramatic gesture was needed to convince the Akron residents that Beloit was the place for them.

Our opportunity came soon. One of the group members had not been able to make the trip to Beloit with his wife because they had recently had a new baby boy. As a result, negotiations were delayed indefinitely. To break the deadlock, I chartered a corporate airplane and flew our search committee and their wives to Akron for a full day of interviews and discussions. Since the candidate couldn't come to Beloit, we brought Beloit to the candidate. After a long afternoon of interviews with residency program directors, the prospective physicians, and a wonderful evening of socializing with our families, an agreement was reached.

I still remember getting back on the plane at 1 a.m. in Akron and announcing to the search committee that we had a signed contract. I purchased a bottle of Dom Perignon at the restaurant and had it placed in a doggie bag for a celebration on the way home. As the chartered plane taxied to the runway, the champagne was uncorked and a toast was offered to our first big success. Nine months after giving our contract group notice, Beloit had its first group of emergency medicine specialists. The flight back to Beloit with a signed letter of intent was one of the highlights of the turnaround and our first big success.

JOINING THE BIG TIME

Beloit's hospital out-migration numbers made it clear that most local residents leaving the community for healthcare were going to one of three tertiary hospitals in a nearby northern Illinois city. Out-migration to those hospitals had a negative secondary effect on primary care business. For example, when a patient was referred to a competing tertiary hospital for heart surgery, neonatal care or other tertiary services, families tended to utilize the tertiary hospitals for primary care. As a result, the more tertiary business we lost, the more primary care business we lost too. The tertiary hospitals were only about a 20-minute drive from Beloit. It was obvious that people were willing to make the trip even for primary care because they perceived the quality of care was better.

This discovery led us to make a strategic decision of great importance. I felt that the tertiary referral pattern to the three nearby Illinois hospitals needed to be redirected. A tertiary hospital approximately triple the distance was selected. The University of Wisconsin Hospital and Clinics, a major referral center for the midwest, was the obvious choice. The distance factor of 60 miles was great enough so that it was unlikely that primary care would be lost to the extent it had been to the nearby Illinois hospitals. Additionally, the medical capability of the University of Wisconsin Hospital and Clinics was superior to all three nearby tertiary hospitals. The question became, how can the tertiary referral pattern be changed?

As it turned out, the University of Wisconsin Hospital and Clinics was looking for primary care hospitals like ours to affiliate with at the same time that Beloit was determining that a change in referral patterns was in our best interest. University Hospital had established an outreach services department under the leadership of a member of their administrative staff, Peter Pruessing. After several months of discussion and negotiations, an affiliation agreement was signed on March 29, 1985, the fifteenth anniversary of Beloit Memorial Hospital. This was our second big success, and an exciting day. Governor Anthony Earl attended the signing ceremonies and acted as a witness to the agreement. In his remarks he complimented both facilities on the progressive nature of the affiliation and its future implications for Wisconsin.

The affiliation arrangement was a win-win situation. University Hospital was gaining tertiary referrals that before had been going out of state. Beloit Memorial Hospital was gaining the prestige of being associated with a major university medical center, as well as clinical services in subspecialty areas that Beloit was not large enough to attract. After the affiliation arrangement was finalized, Beloit began getting regular visits from university subspecialists who conducted clinics right in the hospital in rehabilitation medicine, sports medicine, oncology and allergy. Although Beloit was not large enough to attract specialists in these areas, our community did have individuals who needed those specialists. Before the affiliation they had no choice but to travel long distances to obtain needed care. The new University affiliation gave us the ability to service those patient's needs right in our own community.

In addition to the clinical benefits of the affiliation, University Hospital was also able to provide management support. This came in the form of providing temporary supervisors for departments when recruiting was underway and technical assistance in areas where our expertise was limited. All in all, both parties benefited from this unique partnership. The signing of the affiliation agreement was our second big strategic slate success.

HELP WANTED: MORE LOCAL SPECIALISTS

Declining inpatient business and market research studies confirmed that Beloit Memorial Hospital and local physicians were losing more than one-third of community residents to competing hospitals. Lack of physician specialists was a major contributor to this problem. Market research results helped crystalize recruitment efforts by the specialty clinic in Beloit and also stimulated discussion of recruitments in areas that were covered but not satisfactorily. The clinic mounted an aggressive recruiting campaign which yielded a new neurologist and two additional internists within a year. At that point, however, physician recruiting efforts by the clinic stalled.

Two medical specialties were covered by only one individual each, cardiology and urology. Market research confirmed that three-fourths of the cardiology patients in the Beloit community were out-migrating. In addition, the majority of the cardiology cases identified by local family practitioners were being referred out of town, rather than to the clinic cardiologist. This situation had existed for two decades.

The hospital took a leadership role in breaking the cardiology deadlock. The process was started by approaching University of Wisconsin Hospital and asking them to assist the hospital with recruitment of a second cardiologist. As you can imagine, this met with a tremendous amount of local resistance. Many of the local physicians, especially those in the clinic, thought it was inappropriate for the hospital to be involved in deciding how many subspecialists there should be in Beloit. My position was that the hospital had an obligation to participate in that decision since the hospital was losing three-fourths of the local cardiology business to competing hospitals. After several months of name calling and posturing on both sides, the hospital's position prevailed and a new part-time cardiologist was recruited from University of Wisconsin Hospital and Clinics. The new physician joined the staff of the clinic. The recruitment bruised some clinic egos, to be sure. However, the main concern was to increase the coverage availability of cardiology in Beloit. That came at the expense of some hard feelings, but it was well worth it. The final result was that the availability of cardiology doubled and the cardiology out-migration began falling.

A second major physician recruitment battle arose over urology. For more than 20 years one urologist had a local monopoly. This situation, like cardiology, led to a high amount of out-migration. It was complicated by the fact that the urologist took extended vacation periods and refused to recruit a partner or even *locum tenens* coverage while he was away. This led to dissatisfaction both in the community and among local physicians. Everyone was simply putting up with the irritation, rather than facing it head on. The situation created some unusual requests.

One Monday morning I was accosted by an angry general surgeon who was called in to do an emergency urology operation while the urologist was on one of his extended vacations. The surgeon had never performed the repair that an accident victim needed. Transfer was out of the question because of the patient's unstable condition. The surgeon got through the operation by reading a urology text which described the procedure. When the surgeon finished describing his predicament, he asked me to please buy a better book on urology trauma for the library, one that had more pictures and detailed instructions!

After a year of trying to convince the urologist and the clinic where he practiced to recruit a second urologist, I gave up. I announced that the hospital intended to recruit a second urologist to provide adequate coverage for the community, in addition to expanding the medical coverage. That was just the incentive that the clinic needed. It quickly reversed its position and began recruiting a second urologist. In the meantime, the original urologist got mad and quit. Some of his colleagues hypothesized that he intended to quit all along if he didn't get to keep the monopoly. The hospital recruited a *locum tenens* urologist and installed him in the hospital. Although it took more than a year, the final result was that the clinic hired the *locum tenens* urologist permanently, and a second urologist was subsequently recruited. Both the hospital and local referring physicians ultimately benefited. Again, the hospital served as a facilitator in producing a positive recruiting outcome. Along the way, the hospital president lost a few more social invitations from physicians who didn't like the idea that they were no longer in control of physician recruitment.

DAY SURGERY WITH LIGHTNING SPEED

Market research confirmed that the community was upset with the lack of day surgery facilities. Two certificate of need applications for for-profit surgi-centers to be constructed in Beloit were also pending. The threat of losing even more surgery business to a for-profit "doc in the box" convinced us that the hospital had better move with lightning speed.

The high cost of building a separate day surgery facility and the required certificate of need application time convinced us to evaluate other options. A task force consisting of the vice president of nursing, several head nurses and physicians was mobilized to create a solution. Although the hospital was doing a limited amount of outpatient surgery, it was not done in an organized fashion, and it could not be marketed as day surgery to the community.

The task force quickly identified a common sense solution. Approximately 3,000 square feet of underutilized space was available adjacent to the existing surgery suites. By creatively redesigning the space, the task force was able to plan a day surgery facility without having to build any expensive new operating rooms. The design called for reception areas, changing rooms and special recovery areas for day surgery patients. The actual surgery procedures were to be done in the adjacent operating room suites, making better use of their underutilized capacity.

When the facility design was completed, the task force developed fast track procedures to deal with the patient paperwork and ancillary tests. They created a streamlined approach for lab and x-ray exams and simplified the paperwork associated with day surgery procedures for both patients and physicians.

The facility design and new procedures development took 90 days. Inhouse crews completed construction of the reception area, waiting rooms and recovery rooms in only 60 days, at about half the price of using outside contractors. When construction was completed, the unit was dedicated to a retiring surgeon and was an immediate success. Within weeks of its opening, community residents who had been utilizing other hospitals were returning to our day surgery facility.

The William H. Pollard, M.D. Ambulatory Surgery Unit was a tribute to the teamwork of management, physicians, and nurses. They assessed a problem quickly and created a practical solution. It didn't require years of study or hundreds of thousands of dollars to accomplish. The entire project took less than six months and cost less than $50,000. New surgery activity for the hospital paid for the unit's construction within three months of its opening.

NEW EQUIPMENT, NEW ATTITUDES

I remember walking down the hallway in a nursing unit during my first week in Beloit and tripping over a half-filled bucket of water. When I looked up at the ceiling, I noticed a steady drip being collected in the bucket. As I looked down the remainder of the hallway it appeared to be an obstacle course, with a dozen other buckets in various position gathering water dripping from the ceiling. I quickly tracked down the chief engineer and asked him what was going on. He responded that there had not been enough money to fix the roof in recent years. Buckets were less expensive. The resigned way he shrugged his shoulders when I glared at him was indicative of an attitude of resignation. He wanted a good roof, but money to fix it was not forthcoming.

Market research confirmed that the community perceived Beloit as a low-tech hospital. Money became shorter and shorter in supply as the hospital's financial troubles worsened. Little money was spent on facility upkeep and acquiring new equipment. This death spiral continued to the point where the building leaked like a sieve, the parking lot had potholes large enough to swallow compact cars and equipment being used throughout the hospital was behind the times.

To address this strategic slate issue, a task force led by the vice president of support services began to analyze what was necessary to fix the neglected facility and update the medical technology. A hard look at facilities, equipment that was still working but was behind the times and areas where modern technology was totally lacking followed. The discoveries made our heads spin. Anesthesia machines, x-ray machines and operating room tables were more than 15 years old. Although they still worked most of the time, they were certainly not state-of-the-art. A reliance on less than state-of-the-art methodologies to perform diagnostic procedures was the norm. For example, radiology was not using state-of-the-art mammography procedures to diagnose breast cancer. State-of-the-art laboratory equipment to determine toxicity levels of drug overdose victims was lacking.

A general neglect of the building systems and the cosmetic aspects of the hospital was also evident. Roof leaks had damaged ceilings and wall plaster throughout the hospital. The parking lot and sidewalks were in sad shape. The general disrepair of the walls in the public and patient areas was pervasive. This was particularly distressing in light of the fact that Beloit Memorial Hospital was a splendid architectural creation. Fifteen years after its opening, however, it was downright seedy.

Not only were we dealing with equipment and facility deficits—a fatalistic attitude was present as well. Administration, department directors and even physicians had become so discouraged over the past several years that they stopped asking for needed equipment. They figured the money wasn't available, so why ask. Attitudes were addressed first by giving encouragement. Members of administration, middle management and physicians were asked to create comprehensive "wish lists," assuming that funds would magically become available. These wish lists generated extensive requests to upgrade the equipment and facility in virtually every department in the hospital. Using ad hoc groups of physicians and management, the requests were prioritized to differentiate which were the most critical purchases and which could wait another year or two.

As a result of the department by department equipment and facility analysis, the hospital was upgraded considerably. We spent $1.5 million dollars on new equipment and another half million on upgrading the facilities in year two. Although it took approximately 18 months, the hospital received an entire face-lift and moved from a low-tech hospital into the 1980s with an extensive array of new equipment any community hospital would be proud of. Where did the money come from? A one million dollar bequest or a printing press to produce our own cash never materialized. The money came from dramatic improvements in our hospital's financial operation. Every penny saved on operations was reinvested into equipment and facility. All those dollars saved on reusable water pitchers, better negotiated purchasing contracts, management reductions and so on generated cash to refurbish equipment and facilities.

BACK IN THE BLACK AND ON OUR WAY

In year two, after more fine tuning of expenses, the hospital experienced an operating profit of $302,000, the highest in its history. Operating profits, combined with allocation of depreciation funds which had not been fully available previously due to operating losses, were the key to facility and equipment upgrades. Operating expense savings through better purchasing, renegotiated service contracts and improvements in systems enabled us to invest $2 million in equipment and facilities in year two. These financial successes were led by the vice president of financial services, with help from all department directors and vice presidents.

WE MADE IT

By the end of year two, the hospital had succeeded in achieving all six strategic slate goals. The hospital was back

in the black financially. A new group of emergency medicine specialists had moved into the community. An affiliation with University of Wisconsin Hospital and Clinics had
been completed and four new specialists had been recruited
by the clinic. A day surgery facility was up and running.
Everywhere one looked new high tech equipment and improved facilities were in place. All of our listening strategies
and corporate value progress had changed the attitudes of
employees and improved responsiveness to our customers.

At end of year two, everyone felt great. Most of the
management staff stopped answering ads for positions in
other hospitals. Success was celebrated at the end of the
year and the hospital began to contemplate its future. To
even think about the future was a major step forward. Day-
to-day survival was no longer the dominant issue.

Before talking about the recovery process in year three,
however, one more chapter is necessary. Until this point,
each chapter has ended with brief lessons of hindsight. But
to write of the hindsight lessons learned in completing strategic slate goals requires more than a paragraph or two. It
deserves an entire chapter.

CHAPTER FIFTEEN

Bruised but Undaunted

*T*WENTY YEARS AGO spin train-
ing was part of the program for flight instruction for private
pilots. If you are not familiar with spins, let me assure you
they can be terrifying. First the airplane is pointed nearly
straight up while engine power is reduced. The plane then
stalls, pitching nose down toward earth. To induce the plane
into a spin, a hard left or right turn is executed at the moment it stalls. The plane then plunges nearly straight down,
spinning so fast the world below appears as a blur.

During the turnaround I had a recurring nightmare
which recalled my early flight training. I dreamed I was in a
plane spinning out of control. Everything I tried to make the
plane recover failed. Unlike flight training, the plane just
kept spinning out of control and plummeting straight down.
I always awoke just as the plane crashed. I recall this story
here because there are definitely times in a turnaround
when the leader feels things are out of control, and nothing
he does can stop the inevitable crash. Although we never
crashed there were many near misses and plenty of times
when I thought mistakes were going to finish us off.

THE EMERGENCY ROOM DISASTER

Recruiting an entirely new group of emergency room physicians was not easy. Although the hospital succeeded, there were many difficulties along the way. The first problem came when it was realized that the engagement of a physician search firm to recruit the chief of emergency medicine was not going to produce results. The comfort initially felt upon hiring a nationally known firm evaporated when the few candidates they presented neither met our recruitment specifications nor were the caliber of physicians we wanted joining our staff. After some frustrating meetings, the search firm was fired. The hospital decided to go it alone, recruiting the chief and staff physicians. After that decision, there was no one to blame for failure but ourselves.

The quality of emergency room physician coverage was not that good to begin with, as our community had clearly told us. While recruiting to replace the contract group was underway, quality got worse. Since the contract group knew that the relationship was going to be short term, existing physicians quickly found other jobs. This left us with increasingly short-tenured and inexperienced physicians in our emergency room. In the last four months of the contract, sixteen different physicians covered the emergency room. That doesn't count one who was rejected because she refused to start her shift unless the hospital provided her with free valium. Although the contract company tried valiantly to provide adequate coverage, the quality of physicians went from bad to worse. The community noticed and began complaining even more about emergency room quality. I didn't think it could get much worse. I was wrong.

At the same time, our attending physicians got more upset about the ER coverage too. The emergency room physician short termers were referring more patients out of the emergency room because they didn't have enough time or interest to get acquainted with our attendings' capabilities. Increased transfers decreased business for attending physicians and drove our already low inpatient census to record depths. Some of the more senior attendings began recalling the old days 10 years previously when they had to cover the emergency room themselves. As the situation deteriorated, some attendings became totally convinced that they were going to have to cover the emergency room again, and soon. They weren't pleased at the prospect, to say the least.

The disruption made the emergency room situation worse in the short run in order to achieve a longer run improvement. It was much easier for us to live with the bad situation after the new group had signed their contract. But there was a four month lag between the time when the recruitment had been completed and when the new group finished their residency and moved to Beloit. During that time our emergency room service deteriorated further and tempers were flaring daily. It is a good thing that the recruitment was finished when it was. If it had taken much longer, the vice presidents and I would have been run out of town by an angry community and physicians for taking a bad situation and making it worse. The moral of the story is this—if you're going to make a bold move like recruiting a whole group of emergency room physicians, you better deliver or update your résumé.

IF YOU DON'T SUCCEED, TRY AGAIN

The affiliation with the University of Wisconsin Hospital and Clinics was not without its problems either. Although both hospitals gained from the relationship, along the way it was learned that good communication is essential in achieving desired results.

This lesson was learned the hard way with the introduction of a visiting oncology coverage. This service was set up to have an oncologist see patients on referral from local physicians every other week. Within the first six weeks it was obvious that the oncologist was not getting many referrals. This angered the visiting oncologist, who took out his frustrations on the local medical community. "How dare they not refer to me, I am a world class oncologist," was his attitude. On the other hand, the attitude of local physicians was, "How dare he ask for my cancer referrals when he is only going to be in town once every two weeks." In hindsight, this arrangement was doomed from the start.

Patients with a confirmed diagnosis of cancer want to be seen by a cancer specialist immediately, not in two weeks. Newly diagnosed cancer patients opted to go to other out-of-town oncologists rather than to wait for the visiting university specialist to visit Beloit every other week.

What the university oncologist did not understand was the need for immediate access by local patients. In hindsight, arrangements should have been made for the University oncologist to see newly diagnosed patients immediately, even if it meant traveling 60 miles to Madison. Newly diagnosed cancer patients are not adverse to driving for an hour if they can be seen in a regional cancer center. After the initial patient workup, the patients could then have been seen on follow up every other week when the visiting University specialist came to Beloit. However, both parties gave up in frustration before that insight came to us. The moral of this story is to think through the referral mechanics more carefully and remember that the psychology of specialty referrals is an important part of the arrangement.

THE HONEYMOON WAS OVER

I was fortunate to have a honeymoon period with physicians which lasted almost to the end of year two. In the beginning, physicians were so grateful that something was being done to rejuvenate the hospital that they were very supportive and even friendly. When my family arrived in Beloit we could not find a house to purchase which was just right for us so we rented. In the months that followed, many physicians kept an eye on the local market for us and eventually one helpful physician told us about an interesting home before it was placed on the market. It was perfect for our needs, and we bought it. Another friendly physician, a sailor, helped locate a mooring for my sailboat at nearby Lake Geneva when I struck out with marina operators. Everyone on the medical staff seemed to go out of their way to make me feel at home.

Honeymoons never last forever. Mine was no exception. In year two I began to impose on physician turf. Battles with the clinic over specialist recruiting brought about positive results for the community, but every fight brought the honeymoon one step closer to ending. Also in year two, I began taking action against several physicians for behavior problems and clinical practice problems. The actions ranged from reprimands to forced resignations. I recall reprimanding one particularly disruptive physician. All CEOs have had experiences with ill-tempered, prima donna physicians. Our worst offender had frequent outbursts against nurses in which he used foul and sometimes sexually explicit language. When I told him I was going to have him arrested for sexual harrassment of the staff the next time he had an outburst, he stopped. But, he started knifing me in the back at every cocktail party in town from that moment on.

Clinical problems with physicians had been largely ignored and tolerated by the previous hospital leadership, just as clinical problems with the staff had been. When I suspended an attending physician for not responding fast enough to a deteriorating ICU patient in the middle of the night physicians began to take notice. They also began coming in promptly when told by the nursing staff that their patients were deteriorating. But I stopped getting dinner invitations to physicians' homes. I wonder why?

The most extreme action taken was to force the resignation of a physician who was clearly not capable of practicing quality medicine. Both administration and physician leadership had been passing the buck for years on this physician. The dallying ended abruptly when the medical staff was given an ultimatum by me to force the resignation of the physician or begin formal proceedings to remove him from the staff. To make a long story short, he resigned after a physician member of the executive committee of the medical staff and I told him he had no choice.

Don't get the wrong idea. For the most part our medical staff was highly competent and hard working. But a few immature and incompetent physicians were present on the staff. I stepped into a leadership vacuum and began dealing with problem physicians. As year two drew to a close, there had been enough confrontations to confirm that the honeymoon was over. What I didn't know then was that more problems with the medical staff were just beginning. Year three was even tougher. The year two confrontations seemed like child's play in hindsight.

THINK BIG

One obvious mistake was made in opening our day surgery unit. It was not designed big enough. Same-day surgery was new to us when the facility was designed. Our thoughts were more focused on retaining existing community business than gaining new surgery business from outside our community. After the unit's opening, it was so successful it was beginning to draw new business from peripheral communities. This new business quickly filled the existing capacity of the unit.

If the unit were being designed all over again, it would be twice the size originally settled for. The unused space was there, but we were not thinking big enough to use it. During a turnaround, our thinking was more about survival than growth. Looking back on it, we should have been more optimistic and designed for future growth, rather than just being preoccupied with survival.

DON'T FORGET THE BEDSIDE STANDS AND LOUNGES

Efforts to upgrade the technology image of the hospital were extremely successful. But more attention should have been paid to the day-to-day low-tech equipment with which patients came into direct contact. The physician and executive decision makers knew it was important to improve the high-tech capability in our laboratory and operating rooms. That was self-evident. However, more thought about the equipment items which interacted directly with patients would have been productive since they influence consumer attitudes directly.

For example, old bedside stands were retained and worn-out side chairs with cigarette holes left in the patient rooms. It should have been recognized that patient room furniture and small equipment like blood pressure units and IV poles were just as important to our image as the high-tech, behind-the-scenes hardware. I will never forget getting a call over my direct hotline from an irate patient who concluded that the hospital was no good just because the wheel kept falling off of the IV pole that she was using. I also will never forget the call from a disgruntled patient who wanted to be transferred to another hospital because he thought our heart monitors were as lousy as the bedside radios, which were cracked and held together with surgical tape and paper clips.

Upgrading high-tech facilities and equipment was critically important. Upgrading the equipment and furniture in direct contact with patients, like bedside stands, IV poles and radios, was also important. More sensitivity to all equipment needs and the influence little things have on forming patient impressions of quality would have a been more balanced approach to upgrading technology in our hospital. Eventually, the little things were taken care of, but not without a few embarrassing moments.

MISTAKES YES, REGRETS NO

Successful turnarounds involve making bold moves in short times. Looking back on it, I have concluded that it is almost impossible to move too fast when making bold moves. It is far better to look back on the first year or two of a turnaround and regret a few missteps than to look back at a perfect track record that was not enough to keep the hospital in business.

Attitudes tend to be fluid in a turnaround. Perhaps people are afraid that the hospital will go bankrupt or be downsized to the point that good physicians and employees would not want to be associated with it. Whatever the reasons, CEOs and top management have a tremendous opportunity for creativity and fast paced results in a turnaround. When things begin to get better, this flexibility diminishes. Leaders willing to move fast and hard will make a few mistakes and learn from them.

The old saying, "Lead, or get the hell out of the way" is very apropos in a turnaround. I might add that a leader in motion is much more difficult to shoot down than one who moves too slowly or is intimidated by making big, high-risk decisions. Mistakes were made in year two, but great successes were achieved too. As the hospital prepared to enter year three it was financially sound, strategic slate problems had been resolved and an effective new management team was eager to show the world just how good they could be at rebuilding a once-struggling hospital.

PART IV

YEAR THREE: RECOVERY

Memorable Moment #4:
"This was one of the most immature acts
I have witnessed as a CEO. It was led by
an especially disruptive physician, the
same one I had threatened earlier with
arrest if he kept swearing at the nurses."

CHAPTER SIXTEEN

Good News, Bad News and High Hopes

*A*S BELOIT MEMORIAL HOSPITAL entered into year three of its turnaround, the news was mostly good. Profits were up, many major problems had been fixed and the staff was responding positively to the new leadership direction. Nevertheless, inpatient activity had continued to drop in year two, just as it had for the preceding six years. A follow up market research study was conducted at the beginning of year three to aid the hospital in formulating strategies to finish the turnaround.

The second comprehensive market research study had three objectives. The first was to determine if there had been any improvements in community perceptions. The second was to check on our competitors' strengths and weaknesses. Finally, the study would guide our final phases of the turnaround and the creation of a strategic plan for the future.

GOOD NEWS FOR A CHANGE

Methodology for the follow up study was similar to the initial one conducted 18 months previously. A combination of focus groups and telephone interviews with 300 community residents was used. The telephone questionnaire was identical to the first survey, except for some additional questions to measure image improvement and advertising awareness.

Results from the focus groups and telephone surveys were very encouraging. They indicated that out-migration had been reduced from 34 percent to 20 percent, a major drop of 14 percent. This finding confirmed what was already known: that Beloit's business was starting to increase in year three. Also, the survey indicated that much improvement had taken place in our community image. Nearly half the community, 42 percent, indicated that there was major or moderate improvement in the hospital during the preceding year. Statistically significant improvements were registered in perceptions of physician quality, nursing care, food, environment and staff attitudes. This was just the good news the hospital needed. It was independent confirmation that all of our efforts on the strategic slate and patient relations programs were actually being noticed by the community.

Good news was received about our advertising programs too. Advertising awareness increased 21 percent due to the "We're Listening" advertising campaign. Specifically, individuals surveyed in both the telephone survey and the focus groups indicated that they liked the large pictures of local residents and the ability to call the hospital president directly.

Some bad news was received, however. The image of our physicians continued to be low. There was no improvement registered in either the focus groups or the telephone surveys on physician image. Comparative community data available through our market research firm suggested that Beloit's physician image was far lower than comparable community hospitals around the country. It was discouraging confirmation that image lags reality. Although a number of new physicians had been added to the staff, they had not had enough exposure in the community nor had they developed enough of a patient base for any real improvements in the overall image of our medical staff.

CHECKING OUT THE OTHER GUYS

At the same time that the follow up survey was being conducted in Beloit, the market research firm was hired to study strengths and weaknesses of competing hospitals. The research was conducted in the communities of the competing hospitals, and was modeled after the research conducted in Beloit. Telephone surveys were conducted as if the competing hospital itself had initiated the study. The results were very enlightening. They showed that the three tertiary hospitals in the major metropolitan community in Illinois all had very strong images—so strong we had no business competing with them head-to-head. On the other hand, in spite of their strong image, the survey showed that if Beloit Memorial Hospital continued improving the quality of services locally there was still a chance to win back our local residents who were commuting south.

We also learned that several nearby community hospitals which had been strong competitors had some weaknesses that could be exploited. These weak areas helped focus our marketing strategies in year three and have begun paying off handsomely as Beloit increases its market share in these nearby communities.

WITCHCRAFT AND PANTY HOSE

While the hospital was busy measuring its progress and determining the strengths and weaknesses of competitors, we tried very hard to encourage our physicians to conduct market research on their own image. It was particularly important for us to convince the clinic to conduct its own market research since our studies confirmed that their image and patient loyalty was weak. The hospital frequently received negative complaints about the clinic's image. Often, my telephone hot line calls were complaints about the clinic accompanied by a plea from a frustrated patient to "Do something about their arrogant attitudes." I certainly tried, but did not succeed in convincing the clinic to do its own research until the matter was brought to a confrontation.

After about a year of cajoling, it appeared that the clinic was never going to conduct its own market research study. Their attitude was that business was great, so why bother finding out what the patients think? I brought the matter to a head at a meeting of the joint conference committee of the medical staff and board. I announced that the hospital was going to commission a market research study on the clinic and publish the results. Overnight, the clinic reversed its position and quickly engaged a market research firm to take a hard look at its own image.

It was interesting to observe the attitudes of various groups of physicians when it came to the subject of market research. Almost without exception, our physicians felt that market research was akin to voodoo medicine. At best, they felt that market research might be helpful in selling more panty hose, but not building up medical practices. There were some differences in attitude among age groups as well. The well-established physicians tended to have less interest in learning what the community thought about them. Their practices were full, they had made their money and they had little interest in learning what their customers felt. On the other hand, some of the younger physicians had less rigid attitudes. Perhaps their practices were not yet full and they had not yet made enough money to be indifferent. For the most part, most of our physicians, young and old, had little interest in market research.

After a grudging start, the clinic did complete a market research study and the results were telling. They discovered that they did indeed have major image problems, particularly in physician support areas. For example, their billing service, scheduling practices and waiting time were judged by their customers to be in need of much improvement. These results were taken to heart by clinic physicians and management. They began aggressively trying to deal with the problems their research had discovered. It took them awhile to get going, but at least they finally got started.

CHARTING THE FINAL COURSE

At the beginning of year three, top management felt a little like the crew of a sailboat rounding Cape Horn and starting the final leg on a round the world cruise. Undaunted by storms and problems which had all been overcome, optimism began to mount. Speculation began that the turnaround started two years earlier might just succeed after all.

After reviewing the follow up market research studies, the vice presidents and I selected three strategies for year three to complete the final phase of Beloit Memorial Hospital's turnaround. It was obvious to us that the hospital, although improving, was still in a precarious position. It was just as obvious that the cohesiveness which was so helpful in getting everyone to work together harmoniously in a crisis was beginning to evaporate as improvements in the hospital's finances, image and quality of services became apparent.

For year three, it was decided to focus first on reversing the six-year slide in inpatient business. If that trend could be reversed, it would be obvious to everyone that Beloit Memorial Hospital was in a growth mode, rather than a downsizing mode. Along with this goal, it was decided to produce a substantial amount of new revenue dollars through activity increases, not price increases. If successful, this strategy would clearly prove that Beloit Memorial Hospital was capable of regaining market share in its own community.

A second major focus was related to the image and quality of Beloit Memorial Hospital's medical staff. The single greatest factor in determining the hospital's future success would be the image and quality of our physicians. Not that food, nursing attitudes and high-tech equipment are unimportant. But physician image and quality are more important. No one ever traveled to the Mayo Clinic in Rochester, Minnesota, because the food is good. Physician image and quality draw patients there. Since many of our physicians were resistent to marketing concepts, it was decided that the hospital would have to play a role in improving physicians' image.

The third focus was to begin looking toward the future. The vice presidents and I were committed to have year three be the last year of the turnaround. It was felt that the final phases of the turnaround should include a transition to the future. The creation of a strategic plan was undertaken as the final goal for year three. Looking back on our deliberations at the beginning of year three, I'm still amazed that we never considered the possibility that year three strategies would fail and that the strategic plan would be useless. With two successful years under our belts, the management team was convinced that everything would turn out well. We were almost right.

WHAT ABOUT MORALE?

Ask any general which is more important, weapons superiority or troop morale, and he will say morale without hesitation. In year three, employee morale was soaring. Participation in hospital functions like picnics and Christmas parties broke new records. Employees were doing a wonderful job with patients at the bedside, which was confirmed by numerous letters and positive calls on my hotline. I was especially proud of the nursing staff. Some nurses even began making home visits to former patients after discharge to make sure they were doing O.K. It was a tremendous lift for management to see the staff so high as we entered the final phase of Beloit's turnaround.

LESSONS OF HINDSIGHT

If the opportunity presented itself to go back and undo the timing of the physician market research, I definitely would have gotten more aggressive with our physicians earlier. I tried unsuccessfully for a year to get them to do their own market research. If I were doing it over again, I would have threatened them with doing it ourselves within the first three months and have gotten it over with. The faster the physicians began improving their image, the faster the hospital's image recovery proceeded. A tougher stance with the physicians sooner would have probably put us six months ahead in completing the turnaround.

CHAPTER SEVENTEEN

Generating New Revenue

IN YEAR THREE, the financial
strategy of Beloit Memorial Hospital switched from reducing operating costs to creating new sources of revenue. It is
far easier to reduce operating costs through improved effi-
ciencies than it is to create new revenues. Operating expenses were successfully reduced in year one and year two
in order to return to profitability. The next step was to maintain our expense reduction successes while improving
profits through new sources of revenue.

A LOFTY GOAL

In order to put substance into our strategy of creating new
revenue, the hospital board and management chose a bold
financial strategy for year three. The decision was made to
forgo price increases during that year. The hospital had been
averaging 11 percent per year price increases since 1978.
The only other time the hospital pursued a zero percent
strategy was out of necessity six years previously. That year
the hospital was denied a price increase by the Wisconsin
Rate Setting Committee, and the results were disastrous. The
hospital had its largest operating losses in its history, nearly
$800,000. The following year, it implemented a 20 percent

price increase and still experienced operating losses in excess of $500,000. The proposal to forgo a price increase as part of the turnaround strategy was met with some degree of skepticism by the hospital board. However, it was decided to proceed with the understanding that the board would reconsider in the event the hospital began experiencing major operating losses.

This bold strategy required that the hospital develop approximately one million dollars in new revenue through activity increases in inpatient and outpatient services in year three to break even. At a time when nearly all hospitals in Wisconsin and throughout the country were experiencing declines in inpatient activity, and only moderate growth in outpatient activity, this was a bold move. The management staff, including department directors and vice presidents created a two-fold approach to accomplish our goal of one million dollars in new revenue. The first called for development of completely new services and programs. The second called for increasing activity in the existing services. Results in both areas were successful beyond our most optimistic plans.

WIN/WIN PROJECTS

In developing strategies to create new revenue through new services, the urge was resisted to get into totally new lines of business. It is in vogue these days for hospitals to get into separate lines of business, sometimes related and sometimes not related to the core hospital business. This strategy was not pursued in Beloit. This decision came partly as a result of my conservatism, and partly as a result of not wanting to diversify until it was absolutely certain that our core business was running as well as it should be. Our new activity strategies were created from existing strengths rather than totally new ventures.

Our first new service ventures came as a result of our affiliation agreement with University of Wisconsin Hospital and Clinics. Through the affiliation, visiting subspecialists began conducting outpatient clinics in unused space at the hospital. Initially, these clinics involved allergy and immunology and rehabilitation medicine. By setting up separate clinic space for the allergists and rehabilitation specialists, the hospital was able to develop both office visit revenue and ancillary service revenue from laboratory, x-ray and respiratory therapy, which came as a result of conducting the clinics. This new service was gratifying from both the financial point of view and a community service point of view. The revenue produced was virtually all profit. There was very little cost associated with conducting these clinics. From a community standpoint, new subspecialty medical services were being offered without the requirement of recruiting full-time physicians. It was a win/win situation for the hospital and the community.

Our day surgery program was also a major financial success in year three. With the introduction of this service, the hospital quickly began getting back surgery patients who were previously leaving the community to nearby day surgery facilities. Again, because existing space and staff were utilized, there were virtually no new operating expenses associated with this business. Nearly all the new revenue produced was profit. Again, it was a win/win situation. The hospital was producing new revenue and profits, and residents of the community were getting a service locally that previously they had to travel long distances to obtain.

The next venture was our first attempt at creating an off-site service. Our excellent physical therapy department was teamed with a sports medicine specialist through our affiliation agreement with the University of Wisconsin Hospital and Clinics to create a Sports Medicine Center. This new service was developed entirely on the initiative of our entrepreneurially minded department director for physical medicine. She researched the revenue and cost potential for this service, prepared business projections and was able to convince her vice president and me that this new service was worth a try. She even found an excellent site six blocks from the hospital.

It took only eight weeks from initial concept presentation to opening the Sports Medicine Center. The Center was an immediate success. It began producing new revenue and new profits virtually the day it opened. It was interesting to learn just why we were obtaining so much new business. After several months of operation, it was learned that individuals who utilized the Sports Medicine Center were individuals who did not want the hassles of visiting a hospital physical therapy department. The customers for the Sports Medicine Center were active and relatively healthy people with a minor limiting injury. These customers chose to use the convenient Sports Medicine Center to maintain their therapy. Previously, these patients had quickly dropped out of therapy programs that were part of a traditional hospital setting. At the risk of sounding crude, they did not want their therapy in a "down" setting which included elderly stroke patients and accident victims. When given an opportunity to use a service which was closer to a health club atmosphere, they came in droves.

Our next new service focused on senior citizens. They are one customer group that can definitely be shifted from one hospital to another, depending on the level of satisfaction and price of services. With the help of our market research firm, new programs were created aimed at attracting more Medicare business. The program was called "Senior Advantage." Its primary focus was providing support services to senior citizen customers. For example, a counseling service was created to help seniors take care of their hospital and doctor bills so that they would not have to do any of the paperwork. Special parking spaces were provided, special education programs were offered, discounted cafeteria meals were made available and a no waiting policy for admission to the hospital was implemented for them. It took about six months to begin seeing the fruits of this program. By then it was clear the hospital was experiencing dramatic increases in Medicare admissions and a great deal of positive comment from our senior citizen customers.

Our last major new business venture came in the area of contract services to existing community organizations. After evaluating whether or not we should be in the home care, durable medical equipment (DME) and other related businesses it was decided not to enter these businesses directly. Rather, it was decided to create win/win situations with already existing local businesses. For example, there were two excellent home care businesses already serving the needs of our community. However, they were not able to provide sophisticated home services because of their inability to recruit and retain professional staff. We joined forces with both of these organizations to strengthen both their position and our own.

For example, we enabled them to provide physical therapy, occupational therapy, speech therapy and social services to home care patients through subcontracting the professional staff to them. New sources of revenue were created for us since the hospital billed the home care businesses on a per hour basis. This enabled the home care organizations to expand their services and revenue base. It was the best of both worlds for us and for the home care businesses.

Next, the same subcontracting approach was used with local nursing homes. EKG services, x-ray services, laboratory services and so on were subcontracted at a cost far below what these homes could have afforded to offer those services on their own. This created new sources of revenue for us and enabled local nursing homes to provide a higher level of care than was previously possible.

One particularly creative arrangement was developed by our department director of radiology services. He acquired used portable x-ray units and placed them in the nursing homes. Next an on-call system was created so that whenever a nursing home patient needed an x-ray, the hospital technician went to the nursing home, took the x-ray and brought it back to the hospital for interpretion. Previously, when x-rays were needed at a nursing home, the patient had to be placed in an ambulance, driven to the hospital for the x-ray and then returned to the nursing home afterwards. This new arrangement made it far easier on the patients. And x-ray business increased as a consequence of it being more easily available to nursing home patients.

In total, the combination of these new services generated approximately $600,000 in new revenue for Beloit Memorial Hospital in year three.

TREATMENT FIRST, QUESTIONS LATER

The second major new revenue strategy was to increase the business for already existing services. Our efforts were concentrated in six major areas, and were rewarded with the same dramatic increases in revenue experienced for new services. Increases in revenue from existing services came from a combination of improving these services and making them more accessible to the community. We increased volume dramatically by creating new sub-services within existing departments and improving the equipment or facilities of existing services.

The most significant improved service was the emergency room. The recruitment of a new group of emergency medicine residency-trained physicians, coupled with some creative improvements in emergency room procedures, led to significant increases in our business. The new physicians immediately established higher levels of patient care quality. Since our emergency room receives nearly two thousand visits per month, the word quickly got around the community that there were new doctors in town and that they were extremely competent and caring.

The hospital also made several systems changes which were well received in the community. For example, the completion of paperwork was delayed until after care had been rendered. We knew from interviews with emergency room patients that the single greatest irritator is filling out forms and processing paperwork before patients even get to see a physician. The system was reversed, making sure care came first and paperwork later. Additionally, the new physicians began conducting excellent education programs for the paramedics and emergency medical technicians for regional ambulance squads. Almost immediately, ambulances began arriving from communities 10 to 15 miles away that had long ago given up on Beloit Memorial Hospital. The renewed confidence by the paramedics helped greatly to increase emergency room business, at the expense of nearby tertiary hospitals.

Our hospital also began retaining more admissions as a consequence of having the new emergency room physicians. This was due to two circumstances. The previous contract physicians had such high turnover that they never became fully acquainted with the capabilities of the attending medical staff. As a consequence, many patients were transferred to nearby tertiary hospitals who could have been taken care of by our attending physicians. A second factor had to do with the capabilities of the emergency physicians themselves. Since their training included a full range of trauma and emergency medicine services, the hospital was able to accept more patients who were critically ill or injured. A combination of these two circumstances helped us increase our admissions from the emergency department by approximately 15 percent.

Business in the laboratory and radiology departments was increased through a combination of improved equipment and better patient accessibility. For example, new equipment was acquired for the laboratory, which enabled the technicians to do drug level testing on a STAT basis. Previously, nearly all drug overdoses were transferred to tertiary hospitals because of inability to make a prompt diagnosis. The acquisition of the new laboratory technology enabled the emergency room physicians to make the diagnosis and retain nearly all of the drug overdose cases.

In radiology, new equipment was purchased for radiation therapy. This increased referrals into that department by approximately 30 percent. The new cobalt therapy unit attracted more referrals from southern Wisconsin and northern Illinois, outside our normal service area. Other new equipment like state-of-the-art mammography units dramatically increased outpatient activity. Additionally, the radiology department expanded its on-call availability in ultrasound and nuclear medicine, enabling us to handle more patients in the off hours than was previously possible and also reducing the transfers to other hospitals.

The physical medicine department provided a good example of creating new sub-services to increase existing business. A pain management program was created by an interested staff therapist, which enabled us to utilize the department in new ways. The pain management program was one of the most successful new subservices created in year three. Work-hardening programs were created for area industries, which satisified their need to get workers back on the job as quickly as possible and also brought in new physical therapy business for the hospital.

Additionally, the physical medicine department discontinued a part-time speech therapy contract service and hired full-time speech therapists. This created new capacity, which enabled us to sub-contract services to area nursing homes as well as increase referrals from the hospital itself.

Our vascular diagnostic lab became an example of the merits of improving the physical facility and equipment in order to enhance referrals. The vascular laboratory, centered around the capabilities of an excellent vascular surgeon, was given a completely new facility with new non-invasive ultrasound diagnostic equipment. The combination of new facilities and improved equipment enabled this service to expand its patient base and revenue significantly.

SPEND MONEY TO MAKE MONEY

The goal of developing one million dollars of new revenue for year three was aggressive. By the end of year three, that goal had been exceeded by nearly $200,000. In order to accomplish this goal, new programs and enhancements of existing programs were accomplished. In total, approximately $840,000 in expenses were incurred in order to produce new revenue of 1.2 million dollars. That left the hospital with an operating profit of approximately $360,000. Not only was this the highest operating profit in the hospital's history, but it showed that an aggressive program of revenue enhancement can produce excellent operating profits even in the absence of price increases.

The goal to reverse the six-year decline in inpatient activity was achieved in year three. A 5 percent growth in inpatient business was a dramatic and satisfying accomplishment. For the first time in six years, Beloit Memorial Hospital's trends were going up again. More than a few after work toasts marked that milestone.

LESSONS OF HINDSIGHT

On the positive side, we learned that it is possible to instill entrepreneurial spirit in the department director ranks. Their aggressive pursuit of both new business development and increased activity in existing businesses demonstrated that improved profits can come without the necessity of price increases.

On the other hand, there is such a thing as being too successful. Emergency room experiences pointed this out the hard way. The combination of new doctors, less patient paperwork and improved clinical services in the emergency room quickly became known in the community. The resulting increased business brought a great deal of new revenue to the hospital. It also created an entirely new set of problems.

Since the emergency room facility was seventeen years old, the influx of new patients caused an increase in waiting time for minor emergency cases. Also, since such a good job had been done in restoring confidence in the paramedics, more complex cases that previously had been transferred directly to tertiary hospitals began arriving in our emergency room. This increase in complex cases resulted in further slowing down of services for patients with non-critical problems. It quickly became apparent near the end of year three that our physical facility had been outgrown. Plans were then drawn to build an entirely new facility that would enable us to take best advantage of our excellent emergency room physicians, while still providing prompt care for our patients. In hindsight, we were a victim of our own success. The emergency room image lost a little ground in the community because the promptness of service declined when the activity increased dramatically. Perhaps if we had been more optimistic about the success of our emergency medicine services, a new emergency room might have been contemplated sooner.

On a lighter note, I learned that a CEO can be over-enthusiastic if he isn't careful. When designing our senior advantage program, I decided to offer members a 50 percent discount on cafeteria meals, no strings attached. It wasn't long before seniors started coming to the cafeteria in droves. It got so bad that the seniors soon outnumbered employees and physicians. The cafeteria lines stretched so far that employees began spending half of their lunch breaks waiting in line. So much for CEO insight! The problem was fully resolved by changing the hours that seniors used the cafeteria. In the meantime, some employees wondered about the marketing intuition of their leader.

CHAPTER EIGHTEEN

Success Creates New Problems

In year three, it was apparent that Beloit Memorial Hospital was indeed going to be turned around. Success, however, created a completely new set of problems equally as challenging as the circumstances which necessitated the turnaround in the first place.

Management, physicians and employees involved in completing the turnaround were the source of these new problems. The theme was consistent throughout. Relaxation was the culprit. The more it became apparent that Beloit Memorial Hospital was going to survive, the easier it became to become complacent. If this had gone unchecked, perhaps someone else would be writing a book about Beloit Memorial Hospital's second turnaround a few years from now.

NEW CHALLENGES WITH MANAGEMENT

Beloit Memorial Hospital's turnaround began with downsizing management in year one. In year two, half of the remaining management staff was replaced. The challenge for year three was to mold the new managers and those who remained from the previous administration into an effective working team. This was not an easy task. New managers came to us steeped in the cultures of other organizations. Remaining managers at Beloit Memorial Hospital had to unlearn some bad habits of the previous organization's culture. Blending the new managers and the old in a fashion which fostered teamwork required a great deal of time, personal attention and leadership. The investment came first in the form of numerous management development sessions and special department head and administration meetings described previously. Success in building a new and effective management team created two new problems.

Early in year three the first symptoms of relaxation on the part of the management surfaced. It became clearer as the year went on that the more the hospital prospered, the more the management took success for granted. They were relaxing standards for themselves as well as for their staffs. Early successes of some of the revenue producing ventures led to some less well thought out strategies that generated much disappointment when turned down. Without realizing it, the management staff was relaxing attention to the corporate values which had helped Beloit Memorial Hospital succeed in the first place.

Another management problem surfaced in year three. As word of Beloit Memorial Hospital's successful turnaround spread, department directors and vice presidents became the targets for hospital executive search firms. This was ironic. The very success that our managers had produced gained enough notoriety for Beloit Memorial Hospital to have management "raiders" focus on us as the source of talented executives for other troubled hospitals. Although the loss of some talent is inevitable through the years, I saw this as a major threat to the hospital's future success. You can be sure that our fringe benefit program and management pay scales were such that it was very difficult for other hospitals to hire away our best people. As of this writing, the hospital has not lost any key executives, but the risk is always there. I will do everything in my power to keep our superb staff together as long as possible.

MORE MONEY, LESS HASSLES

At the beginning of Beloit Memorial Hospital's turnaround, employees were uniformly apprehensive and willing to do almost anything to save their jobs. Unfortunately, anxiety-induced flexibility does not last forever. Employees had many major adjustments to make during the three year turnaround. Not all of them went smoothly.

It was difficult for some employees to adjust to new work standards. The laissez faire style of management in previous years had led to an environment where discipline was almost nonexistent. For example, one 10-year employee had missed over 200 days of work due to illness, and there was no discipline of any kind for poor attendance. With the implementation of corporate values, a stricter code of discipline was enforced. This meant that disciplines ranging from verbal warnings to terminations were now becoming commonplace for violations of the hospital's corporate values and standards. For the first time, employees were being terminated for such problems as having a poor work ethic, poor quality standards or even poor attendance records. This was especially difficult on the nursing staff, where quality of patient care standards were not well articulated in previous years. For the first time, nurses were disciplined, sometimes terminated, when serious care quality issues were identified. This created an environment of fear and apprehension.

When terminations and suspensions were used, it created an environment where employees began asking themselves, "Who is going to be next?" It took almost a year to work through the various insecurities that were brought about by the increasing use of discipline. One strategy that helped greatly was the publication of completely new disciplinary procedures by the personnel department. They were simple, easy to understand and less subject to interpretation than previous policies. Although employees did not like the fact that discipline was being handed out, when the new policy was explained appropriately, the level of understanding increased to the point where they at least grudgingly accepted the new standards.

Attitude standards were also being enforced. This too created apprehension. The presence of a poor attitude was for the first time considered grounds for discipline, including termination. Since attitudes are very subjective, a great deal of attention had to be placed on educating the department director and vice president staff on identifying attitude problems and dealing with them constructively. Most of these problems were worked through successfully in year two. But in year three, it became evident that employees, like the management staff, were beginning to relax. Now that the crisis of hospital survival was obviously over, the flexibility that employees exhibited to save their hospital became less evident. Like management, employees began taking the hospital's success for granted.

This attitude manifested itself at union contract negotiation time in year three. One-fourth of the hospital's work force, all service employees, is unionized. It was not difficult to negotiate an acceptable contract during the crisis period in year one of our turnaround. At the end of year three, when our financial success was obvious to everyone, negotiating with the union became quite a bit more difficult. It wanted a bigger piece of the pie and could not understand the hospital's need to reinvest profits back into the operation for future growth. It took a great deal of posturing and name calling to finally get an acceptable contract settlement at the end of year three.

HOW QUICKLY THEY FORGET

Physicians were not immune from the relaxation response. It was obvious to them by the beginning of year three that the crisis of the hospital's survival had passed. Their extremely flexible attitudes of the first two years began to harden. During the time the hospital's survival was in question physicians wanted nothing to do with "meddling in management." In fact, they stayed as far away as possible from management decisions.

However, as the hospital's fortunes improved, their attitudes changed. By year three, it began to be commonplace to have fights with physicians over small issues. Also, the centralized authority which had made the turnaround possible began grating on some physicians. That generated the major "Who's in charge?" fights discussed in chapter 20.

The major issue with physicians was that their willingness to accept new ideas and change diminished considerably in the latter phases of the hospital's turnaround. Also, since it was very difficult for physicians to challenge the substance of the hospital's turnaround, they began challenging the style which produced successful results. Physicians who previously wanted nothing to do with management were experts on how and what decisions should be made. All of a sudden physicians overnight became lawyers, interior decorators, personnel specialists and on and on. By the beginning of year three, the honeymoon was clearly over.

THE BOARD WAS NOT IMMUNE

By the beginning of year three, some new problems with the board of trustees also surfaced. In a sense, management was the victim of its own success. As it became clearer and clearer that the hospital was going to survive and prosper, the board, like the medical staff and employees, began showing an interest in getting more involved in operating decisions and details. Some trustees began to question the centralized leadership style which had made the turnaround possible. A few open confrontations at board meetings took place over the authority of the CEO. I was caught completely off guard at one board meeting by a usually quiet member who berated the board for not being more involved in hospital decision making. He got no support from fellow board members, but I was forced to recall that "a CEO's authority is based almost totally on the last financial statement."

The board at this time also began hearing more complaints about management from physicians. As mentioned previously, physicians could not argue with the fact that the hospital was prospering. However, railing against the centralized authority of the hospital CEO, they began doing some behind-the-scenes politicking with board members about my "dictatorship" style of management. A strong leader is very threatening to a medical staff. The medical staff has more access to the board than the CEO due to their sheer numbers. In year three, Beloit had over 50 physicians and 15 board members. Physicians and board members paths crossed continuously on the golf course, at parties and elsewhere. By year three, I saw some evidence of this behind-the-scenes politicking.

My challenge was to focus the board's attention on more long-range issues. This was accomplished through the creation of a new strategic plan, discussed in chapter 19.

NEW PROBLEMS FOR ME TOO

Not even the CEO was immune to the new problems brought about by the hospital's earlier successes. The style of management used during the hospital's turnaround was very autocratic. I judged this to be necessary in light of the laissez faire approach of the previous administration and the need for quick decision making and results. However, with survival ensured, my challenge was the transition into a more teamwork style of management. This cannot be done overnight and represented a major challenge to my leadership.

Another new problem was to keep the organization's passion and momentum going. In the early years of the turnaround, the issue of survival kept the adrenalin flowing and prohibited relaxation. With survival ensured, it is more difficult to sustain positive momentum. Obviously a new set of challenges was required to keep the same level of energy directed to the hospital's future as had been directed to the hospital's survival. A new strategic plan was the vehicle chosen to accomplish this.

Last but not least, my success as the turnaround agent generated many rumors in the community that I would be moving on soon. Some weeks in year three I was asked every day by board members, physicians, employees, community leaders or even the press about how long I planned to stay. Some antagonistic physicians joined in too by starting and promoting the rumors that I would be moving along shortly since the turnaround had been accomplished. These rumors created an environment of uncertainty which did nothing positive for the hospital's future.

LESSONS OF HINDSIGHT

The late Senator George Aikin of Vermont, as blunt and crusty a legislator as ever produced in New England, once said that the way to win the war in Vietnam was to "declare victory and walk away." In sense, that is the lesson of hindsight for this chapter. Success produced a whole new series of problems for our hospital. The most pervasive of these problems was the uniform feeling that the crisis was over and everyone could relax and go back to business as usual. My challenge, as CEO, was to be sure that this did not happen.

The approach to refocus the energy of the various hospital groups was to declare victory and move on. In year three, I made it known that the hospital had been turned around. Though some felt that declaration was premature, no one argued too strenuously. It was time to look to the future.

The biggest joy from turning around an organization comes not from survival, but from making the organization into something to be truly proud of. Creating "Plan 1990" was our way of declaring victory and looking to the future.

CHAPTER NINETEEN

Planning the Future

THE TIMING to complete the new long-range plan for Beloit Memorial Hospital was carefully selected. By the middle of year three, the hospital's finances were stable, activity trends were improving for the first time in six years and my credibility with the board was high. Beloit Memorial Hospital needed a major shove forward to sustain the positive momentum.

I concluded that the hospital's future success was contingent on making critical changes, especially in the medical staff area. Timing was critical. Had I attempted to create a long-range plan earlier, with major implications for the medical staff, my credibility and track record might not have been strong enough to carry it off. On the other hand, had I waited several more years, it might have been too late. Knowing that more controversy was ahead, I initiated the long range planning process.

CONSULTANT VS. INHOUSE PLANNING

The first planning decision was whether to hire an outside consulting firm to do our long-range plan or to do it ourselves. There are many excellent consulting firms available to prepare strategic plans. I felt that the drawbacks of consulting firms were the cost to complete the strategic planning study and the lack of creativity that some of them demonstrate. Also, there is sometimes a lack of ownership among members of the board, medical staff and management when a plan is done by an outside firm.

We elected to complete our long-range plan internally. Along with marketing, I believe the CEO and key board, management and medical staff leaders should provide the vision for charting a hospital's future. It is a job which should not be left to inside staff planners or outside consultants. Several components of the long-range plan were subcontracted to consultants, including demographic projections, market research, medical staff need projections and the architectural plan. But the greater part of the plan was completed by our own internal leaders.

DESIGNING THE PLANNING PROCESS

Assembling the management group to thoroughly review the hospital's performance during the past three years was the starting point. This review included analysis of financial statements, activity trends and market research studies. At the conclusion of this review, the vice presidents and I designed a long-range plan process and presented it to the hospital board. The plan included the following components: SWOT (Strengths, Weaknesses, Opportunities, Threats) analysis; demographic projections; medical needs plan; facility plan; capital equipment plan; financial plan; and new services and program plans.

The plan itself was to be written by the long-range planning committee of the board of trustees, with staff assistance from myself and the vice presidents. A timetable and the plan design were presented to the board planning committee and were approved. The timetable called for Plan 1990 to be completed in 20 weeks. An overview of the planning timetable appears in figure 9.

To complete Plan 1990, the board planning committee was expanded to include several additional members of the medical staff in order to ensure that physicians had suffi-

FIGURE 9

Strategic Plan Timetable

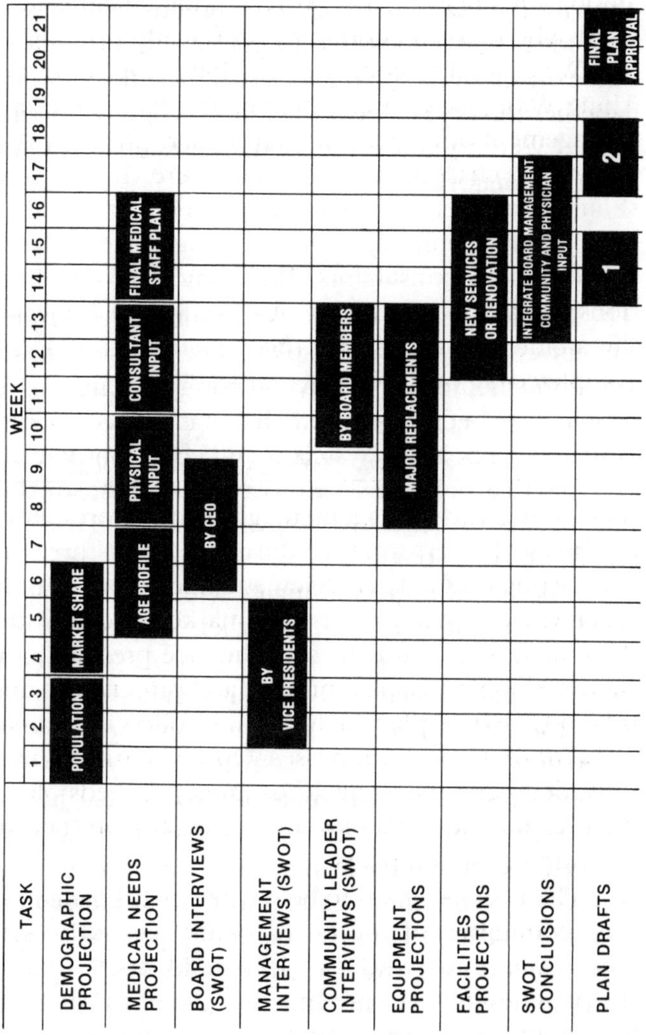

TASK	WEEK																				
	1	2	3	4	5	6	7	8	9	10	11	12	13	14	15	16	17	18	19	20	21
DEMOGRAPHIC PROJECTION	POPULATION			MARKET SHARE																	
MEDICAL NEEDS PROJECTION					AGE PROFILE			PHYSICAL INPUT			CONSULTANT INPUT			FINAL MEDICAL STAFF PLAN							
BOARD INTERVIEWS (SWOT)							BY CEO														
MANAGEMENT INTERVIEWS (SWOT)			BY VICE PRESIDENTS																		
COMMUNITY LEADER INTERVIEWS (SWOT)										BY BOARD MEMBERS											
EQUIPMENT PROJECTIONS									MAJOR REPLACEMENTS												
FACILITIES PROJECTIONS													NEW SERVICES OR RENOVATION								
SWOT CONCLUSIONS														INTEGRATE BOARD MANAGEMENT COMMUNITY AND PHYSICIAN INPUT							
PLAN DRAFTS														1			2		FINAL PLAN APPROVAL		

cient input. Putting several extra physicians on the planning committee was not enough to satisfy some physicians. They thought the entire medical staff should participate. I vetoed that idea. It is impossible to get an entire medical staff to agree on anything. If you asked for a medical staff to vote on whether the sky is blue on a cloudless day, rest assured some would vote no and some would abstain so as not to agree with the majority.

GETTING STARTED

The first job was to design the input gathering process for key groups within the hospital. The decision was made to do a much more extensive input-gathering process than would have been possible with an outside consulting group. Initially, the board, physicians and community leaders were selected to give input. Their assessment of hospital strengths and weaknesses, areas for improvement, and their vision for the future was sought.

I designed a questionnaire with similar questions for each of the three groups, and then assigned responsibility for completing the interviews. The process started with the board. I interviewed each board member personally to review the eight planning questions developed for the questionnaire. I felt it was essential that each board member have an opportunity to participate and to present his or her vision of the hospital's future. Next, the board was utilized to interview community leaders. The planning committee selected 30 community leaders to be interviewed as part of the hospital's long-range planning process. Each board member was assigned two community leaders to interview. A questionnaire similar to the one used with board members was developed and mailed to community leaders in advance. Then, each board member spent approximately ninety minutes with the community leaders interviewing them about the hospital. This proved an excellent way to involve the entire board in the long-range planning process.

Next, members of the medical staff were interviewed by

the vice presidents and me. We each interviewed 10 physicians. Their cooperation was excellent. It would simply not have been possible to interview each physician personally if an outside consultant had been used. Examples of the questions used to gather input from the board, community leaders, and medical staff are provided in Appendix D.

The input approach with the management staff and employees was different. For management, a planning retreat was held where each department head and vice president had an opportunity to present his or her suggestions for how to make Beloit Memorial Hospital the best community hospital in the country. During the retreat suggestions were evaluated and recorded to be integrated with input from other groups. An essay contest was held in which employees were invited to write an essay on how Beloit Memorial Hospital could become the best community hospital in the country by the end of the decade. As an incentive, a vacation in the Bahamas for the winning essay and cash awards for honorable mentions were offered. Much to our delight, there was excellent employee participation, with some extremely well thought out essays which provided valuable insight for the planning process.

PHYSICIANS AND HARDWARE

With the input-gathering process underway our attention was turned to the remaining components of the plan. To assist with developing a medical needs plan an independent consultant was hired to utilize Beloit's population base to determine how many and what types of physicians were needed in the community. Many excellent planning ratios are available from various sources. The consultant utilized these ratios to develop a medical staff configuration which would best meet our community needs in the future. A demographer was also engaged to project Beloit and surrounding community populations through the end of the decade.

An architectural firm was utilized to prepare an updated facilities plan. This facility plan might be characterized as a "quick and dirty" plan, rather than a $200,000, year-long architectural wonder. The architect evaluated existing departmental relationships and identified major problem areas. He also evaluated various facility and new service options being considered as part of the planning process and estimated implementation costs. Simultaneously, physicians, department directors and vice presidents were identifying major equipment needs through the end of the decade. Existing equipment and facilities were analyzed very carefully, and major facility and equipment replacement needs identified.

Input gathering took approximately 10 weeks. After summarizing the input from various interest groups, there was a consensus about the hospital's strengths and weaknesses and a wide range of options in terms of new programs and facilities desired by these groups. The next step was to make some preliminary decisions about which options represented the board's desire for the hospital's future. To facilitate these decisions, a summary of the hospital's strengths and weaknesses and program options was prepared for consideration by the full board of trustees.

MAKING THE PRELIMINARY DECISIONS

As part of our timetable, a special board meeting was planned for halfway through the planning process to evaluate major options. This meeting was held, with several additional members of the ad hoc planning committee present. Two sets of decisions were needed. First, the list of approximately 20 new program options needed to be narrowed to a more manageable size. Beloit Memorial Hospital could not be all things to all people. Our future focus had to be narrowed. Second, a major decision about how to approach medical staff problem issues had to be made. According to the input gathered in the planning process the medical staff's image was the hospital's major weakness. Exactly how to go about changing that situation presented some interesting options.

I prepared a set of working papers for each of these two major decisions and presented them to a special meeting of the full board. At the conclusion of the first discussion, the list of 15 options was narrowed to seven. The planning committee was then charged with further developing these seven new program options for integration into the hospital's long-range plan.

With reference to the second decision item, dealing with the medical staff, there was a lively and spirited debate. At the end of that debate, the board concluded it would take a more active role in the future in determining the size, composition and activities of the hospital's medical staff. This was a profound departure from the past. Our hospital, like many around the country, had taken a hands off approach and let the medical staff determine its own levels of quantity and quality. Beloit's board decided this no longer would be appropriate. It decided that the long-range plan would include a medical needs plan which would determine the board's expectations for various specialties and quality levels for future physician recruiting. Additionally—and this was a departure of major significance—it decided that the long-range planning process would include market research studies on local physicians' image and requirements for improvement of that image over time.

As you might imagine, those decisions produced the proverbial "shots heard around the world" from physicians. The medical staff began to suspect they had lost control over the hospital's major decisions. They didn't cherish the thought. They wondered who was in charge. More on that in the next chapter.

THREE TIMES A CHARM

The long-range planning schedule called for three drafts of Plan 1990. The first draft was completed shortly after the full board decided on options for new programs and its future approach to the medical staff. This draft was presented to the planning committee for review 14 weeks into the process. At this point, the plan still had several options to be decided upon and there was more lively debate in the planning committee. At the same time, physicians who had not been personally involved in the planning process were debating the plan's content and merit. A gigantic "Who's in charge?" fight was brewing.

After evaluating input from all planning committee members, the second draft was completed. After the second draft was reviewed by the planning committee, I convened a special meeting of the medical staff to review its contents. This meeting diffused most remaining negative sentiment on the part of the medical staff. That special meeting was well-attended and no objections were raised, even though several weeks earlier the plan was being soundly roasted by members of the medical staff.

A third and final draft of the plan was written and approved for adoption by the long-range planning committee, on schedule. That ended 20 weeks of effort by a dedicated group of board members, physicians and management. There was a tremendous sense of ownership of the plan, because we had essentially done it ourselves, with little outside assistance except in technical areas. Shortly thereafter, the plan was adopted by the full board and then distributed to board members, physicians, management and employees.

The significance of Plan 1990 is twofold. First, it confirmed that the hospital's turnaround was over and that attention was going to be focused on future growth rather than survival. Second, Plan 1990 presented management with a new set of goals, even more challenging than the turnaround.

LESSONS OF HINDSIGHT

One major error was made in our long-range planning process. It applied to the medical staff. Although several physician non-board members were placed on the long-range planning committee, it proved to be not enough. After the full board's initial decisions on the major options, word got back to the medical staff that the hospital was planning some major new programs which would negatively influence the medical staff. Although that was not in fact true, it nevertheless generated tremendous amount of heat and very little light.

In hindsight, this could have been avoided. A special meeting of the full medical staff should have been built into the planning process to review plan options before presenting them to the full board. In that way, the medical staff would have had an opportunity to comment and give input before I presented the decision options to the board. Communicating with the full medical staff, rather than just a few members of the planning committee might have dampened some of the false rumors and ensuing hard feelings.

It also points out the danger of doing a long-range plan internally. With an outside consulting firm handling the process, its easy to blame them when things go astray. Since I was leading the planning process personally, I took the full brunt of the negative medical staff feelings toward certain aspects of the plan. I still think doing the plan internally was right. However, the next time I will be certain that one more meeting with the full medical staff gets added to the schedule to minimize the false rumors and hard feelings.

CHAPTER TWENTY

Who Is in Charge?

W_{HO} RUNS THIS PLACE anyway? The board, CEO or the medical staff? CEO's have fought "Who's in charge?" battles many times in many hospitals throughout the country. Sometimes they win and sometimes not. In our case, the "Who's in charge?" battle began building in year two and culminated in year three of the turnaround. By the time it really got hot I was comfortable that the hospital's image had improved greatly, its finances were in good shape and its activity levels moving upward again after six years of decline. On the other hand, I was equally confident that moving the hospital ahead was contingent on major changes in the medical staff. Specifically, future progress was contingent on major improvements in the clinic, which dominated the medical community in Beloit.

Over the years, it appeared to me that there was a much too comfortable relationship between the hospital and the clinic. This easy relationship benefited neither party. The hospital had not been demanding toward the clinic or its physicians. As a consequence, the number of specialists was insufficient to meet the needs of the community. In addition, the quality and poor attitudes of some specialists tended to create a negative perception of the clinic as a

whole. This contributed to an overly high out-migration for
physician related reasons. The clinic had only a 60 percent
market share in Beloit, even though it was the only one in
town providing specialty medicine services. Not very impressive.

On the other hand, the clinic had not been very aggressive toward the hospital, either. The clinic had not developed much in the way of ancillary services to compete with
the hospital. They even used this lack of aggressiveness to
their advantage whenever a confrontation was brewing between the hospital and the clinic. For example, when the
clinic didn't like something the hospital was doing, they
threatened to add ancillary services and take revenue away
from the hospital. It was almost a standing joke. The attitude was, "If you make us mad, we will put an ultrasound
machine in and take away an important source of revenue
and profit." The hospital had always folded under this
threat. It was a cowardly position which caused the clinic to
become more and more arrogant. It was controlling the hospital and medical care in the community. The clinic physicians did a poor job on the former and only a mediocre job
on the latter.

The outcome of this too comfortable relationship was
bad for the clinic, the hospital and the community. The lack
of aggressiveness on the part of the hospital toward the
clinic yielded a less than adequate number of specialists.
The community suffered the consequences, since patients
had to leave town for needed specialty care. It was a disgrace that no oncology or neurology service was available,
and only questionable coverage was available in cardiology,
urology and dermatology, to name just a few. The hospital
suffered, too, since the number of people out-migrating had
reduced revenues to the point where its survival was in
question.

BUILD-UP

The build-up of tensions leading to the "Who's in charge?"
fight took about a year. During year two, I had forced the is-

sue on several specialty recruitments, and had begun disciplining physicians for behavior and clinical problems. The opening salvo of the war came when the hospital recruited the first hospital-based specialist. Early in year three, the hospital made a commitment to develop a million dollar invasive cardiology facility. The clinic agreed to recruit only one of the two invasive cardiologists that the hospital felt was necessary to obtain maximum benefit from this new facility. I made it known that this was unacceptable. With ample warning, I began recruiting a second invasive cardiologist to be based at the hospital, rather than the clinic.

This was a major departure from past practice. Previously all specialists had been based at the clinic. Although the clinic was well-informed about my recruiting intentions, they paid no attention until the final candidate was nearly on board. Then, it really hit the fan. Many clinic members mobilized to stop the recruitment effort. They politicked with board members, applied pressure on me and tried to convince the prospective cardiologist that she was not welcome in the community. A physician board member, also a member of the clinic, politicked hard to get the recruitment stopped. To add insult to injury, I had recommended that this physician be appointed to the board, thinking that he would be an objective and rational influence. Was I ever wrong! The recruitment became a very emotional issue, and several physicians tried to get me fired by cornering board members and letting them know that my aggressive management style was incompatible with harmonious medical staff relations.

This first battle raged for about a month. When it was over I had successfully completed the recruitment of the hospital-based cardiologist, in spite of the clinic's objections. The support of the board as well as the non-clinic family physicians was instrumental in completing this recruitment. It was the first case in which the hospital had taken a strong anti-clinic stand for the benefit of the community. I was gratified with the outcome. The board's support was crucial. Their attitude was that medical staff relations should be allowed to suffer in the short run in order to correct medical coverage problems which would serve the community better in the long run.

However, tensions increased significantly between myself and the clinic after that recruitment. The next step in the tension build-up came as part of the medical staff's review and updating of its bylaws. As a protest to the physician consultant engaged to help update the bylaws, several clinic members engineered a walkout during a medical staff meeting. This was one of the most immature acts I have witnessed as a CEO. It was led by an especially disruptive physician—the same one I had threatened earlier with arrest if he kept swearing at the nurses. The walkout had a predictable result. It drew the board, management and even employees into the battle. For several weeks the tensions escalated out of control.

THE BIG FIGHT

The clinic-engineered walkout occurred simultaneously with completion of the first draft of the long-range plan. A number of special physician meetings were held, some clandestine, to discuss the hospital's alleged plan "to get the medical staff." Although the issues were clouded with emotions and flaring tempers, the real issue was who was going to be in charge of the medical community, the board or the clinic. The balance of power had always rested with the clinic. The hospital had always deferred to its threats. Now, for the first time, the hospital CEO was leading the charge to change the balance of power. And the board was strongly supporting the CEO's efforts.

Until year three, turnaround efforts had not really negatively impacted the medical staff. Quite to the contrary, most of the successful new ventures created new sources of revenue for physicians and created a better-equipped hospital for them to practice medicine in. However, some clinic physicians felt the long-range plan was a significant threat to their independence. It was not. It was an effort on the part of the hospital board and me to set some definitive standards for the medical staff. But for some of the physicians on our staff, standard is a dirty word. The long-range plan did indeed call for the recruitment of specified numbers of physicians, rather than leaving it totally up to the clinic as had been the previous practice. In addition, the long-range plan called for a comprehensive image study of all physician groups within the community, and it further called for specific improvements in the image over time. Without question, the long-range plan was very aggressive. It changed the balance of power. The board set overall medical policy, rather than physicians. A new concept in Beloit.

THE FIRESTORM

During the month or so following the infamous walkout, there were many harsh words for the hospital CEO. Physicians could not attack the substance of the hospital's turnaround, so they spent a great deal of time attacking me personally. Physicians began asserting that the same turnaround results could have been accomplished with a less confrontational leadership style. I did not care much for their style either.

Several vocal physicians led an effort to lobby the hospital board to get me fired. When that accomplished no immediate results, they began spreading rumors in the community that I was going to leave because physicians were making life miserable for me. Half of that rumor was true. The stronger the criticisms became, the more evident it became that the anti-CEO charge was being led by a few insecure physicians rather than the whole medical staff. It amazed me how much passion a few disgruntled physicians could stir up. In addition to threatening to get me fired, some physicians even went so far as to threaten to drive the hospital census down to bring the hospital to its knees.

As you might imagine, that threat did not help their cause with the hospital board. Although the census did fluctuate downward during this troubled period, I still do not

believe that our physicians lacked character to the extent
that they would decrease the hospital's census just to make a
point. But who knows? Additionally, the clinic began threatening again to take away ancillary business as they had in
the past. Much to their surprise, I told them to go ahead. I
felt very comfortable competing with them on any basis. I
did not immediately contract diarrhea and cave in to their
threats. That took some of the wind out of their sails.

THE AFTERMATH

Although I was the subject of many personal and professional attacks by certain physicians during the hottest of the
"Who's in charge?" battle, I kept my cool. Communicating
was the best way to deal with their passion. In the midst of
the worst of the battle I attended a clinic board meeting to
review the elements of the long-range plan for them.

Although I had to listen to a long diatribe of putdowns
before I was able to speak, some clinic members listened. In
addition, a special medical staff meeting in which all physicians were invited to preview the long-range plan draft
helped.

Two things turned the tide in the "Who's in charge?"
battle. First, it became apparent to some physicians, even inside the clinic, that their anti-administration colleagues had
gone too far. Moderate physicians began reminding their
colleagues that I had indeed led the hospital's turnaround.
Regardless of the style in which that turnaround was
achieved, they felt I deserved credit for accomplishing it.
Second, some of the non-clinic physicians began being vocal against clinic physician efforts to discredit me and the
hospital's long-range plan. Keeping my cool and not react-
ing to the attacks helped to diffuse the situation as well. Another thing helped. I never got mad in public. No matter
how insulting physicians became, I did not respond in kind.
My coolness under attack drove them crazy. Behind closed
doors, however, I made a point of telling several of them
what I thought of their tactics. I think I may even have ex-

panded the vocabulary of a few detractors during these woodshed sessions.

No question about it, a major "Who's in charge?" battle is hard on the gastric mucosa of any CEO. Virtually all of the social contact I had with physicians before the battle ceased afterward. Many of those I had considered friends deserted me in the midst of the battle until they saw which way the wind was blowing. All except six, that is. They had the courage to stand up for me, even in clinic meetings when their colleagues were burning me in effigy. Afterwards, some physicians cautiously re-established some of their old ties. I was grateful to those few physicians who, risking the rebuke of their peers, stood up for me and what was right during the battle. There weren't very many, though.

THE FINAL OUTCOME

In the final analysis, the hospital board won the "Who's in charge?" battle. The board adopted Plan 1990, which specified a medical development plan and establishment of image standards for the medical staff. There were some residual hard feelings, and there probably always will be as a result of this battle. On the other hand, the responsibility for doing what is right for the community now clearly rests with the board, where it belongs. The ability of individual physicians or even a large clinic to dominate medical decision-making policy no longer exists. Beloit will benefit, and even those physicians who fought hard against the policy will benefit in the long run.

LESSONS OF HINDSIGHT

Three items are important to prevail in any CEO/physician "Who's in charge?" battle: Timing, timing and timing. I picked the timing very carefully for my "Who's in charge?" battle. I am certain timing enhanced my ability to succeed. Had I chosen to fight earlier, the hospital would not have been in as good shape as it was, and my credibility would not have been as high. Had I waited another year or so, physicians' attitudes might have been so set in stone that they would have prevailed.

Another important aspect of timing is managing other related issues and confrontations. A wise person once said that you can get some of the people mad at you some of the time, but avoid getting all the people mad at you at once. I chose the time for my "Who's in charge?" fight to be one when no other group would be confronting me while the physician battle was going on.

A parting word of advice for a CEO who finds himself faced with a "Who's in charge?" battle. Follow your conscience. I decided in year three that I had led the hospital as far as I could take it without a major confrontation with physicians. I decided, even before beginning the long-range planning process, that dealing with medical staff problems was worth getting fired for. I believe the board and medical staff understood this. If an individual is not willing to be fired over a matter of professional principle, he has no right to the CEO's chair.

The approval of the hospital's long-range plan and the winning of the "Who's in charge?" fight was truly the end of our hospital's turnaround. The hospital was in a position to decide its destiny again. It had a long-range plan which defined its destiny in concrete terms. As year three drew to a close, I felt very good about the prospects for Beloit Memorial Hospital's future. There was another plus to be happy about as well. Since I stopped getting Christmas cards and social invitations from physicians that year it cut down on my postage and entertainment expenses the following year.

Hindsight Revisited

TURNAROUNDS are tremendous opportunities. Look at Chrysler Corporation. It proved a company in trouble can come back stronger than ever. Turnarounds are learning experiences for all parties. Beloit's key lesson was that teamwork and strong leadership can create order out of chaos and excellence out of mediocrity.

From the CEO's perspective, common sense, persistence and a driving passion to succeed are far more important than high-priced consultants, a Harvard Business School education or stopwatch-wielding industrial engineers. A strong stomach doesn't hurt either.

STATESMEN NEED NOT APPLY

The strategies utilized to turn Beloit Memorial Hospital into a successful and growing organization can be applied to any hospital, large or small. Additionally, the common sense management approaches which were useful in turning around Beloit Memorial Hospital can be applied to hospitals that desire to be more competitive, more profitable and more customer oriented.

The first step in a turnaround, or major improvement in a stagnant hospital, is recognizing that change is needed. This recognition must begin with the Board. It may cause a change in leadership, or it may mean renewed commitment to an existing leader. Whichever is the case, the turnaround leader needs absolute support from his board.

After recognition that improvement and change are necessary, the full commitment of the CEO to be the change agent is needed. The CEO must recognize that the turnaround will require his full intellectual commitment. There will be little time for Rotary meetings and committee memberships in the American Hospital Association if a turnaround is to succeed. The CEO who sees himself as an "outside man" or health statesmen has no business attempting a turnaround. The turnaround CEO must also be a risk taker, prepared to make bold moves with uncertain outcomes.

FIRST TASKS

Our experience indicates that it is vital to focus on finances early in a hospital turnaround. The reduction of expenses, beginning with management expenses and staff expenses, followed by more intelligent and aggressive purchasing of supplies, services and systems is critical.

If financial problems are not resolved early, there may be no organization left to turn around. Early emphasis should be on cost control, rather than revenue increases. We were particularly reluctant to increase revenue through price increases. To me, that would have been the equivalent of going duck hunting with a Uzi submachine gun. Effective, but not quite fair.

While financial problems are being resolved, it is absolutely vital to "get the picture." Our experiences suggest that getting the most accurate picture involves hiring an outside market research consultant. This requires money up front. That may be difficult while the hospital is facing financial problems. But market research money invested during the early days of a turnaround can be the best investment in the hospital's future. The effective turnaround leader must also be prepared to listen carefully to market research results. Getting defensive and pointing fingers will not help. Listening and formulating strategies to resolve identified problems is much more productive.

A turnaround is a short-term endeavor. Through the use of strategic slates, our energies were focused on the short term. Planning for the distant future was avoided. Creating a five- or ten-year long-range plan in the midst of a turnaround is a contradiction in strategies. Also, focusing on the short term and resolution of problems involves commitment of resources. This, too, may be difficult when the hospital is facing financial problems. However, risks must be taken and money spent in order to make needed improvements. We certainly confirmed that hypothesis by doing things such as chartering airplanes for physician recruitment. The rewards for those types of investments far outweighed the costs.

CREATING A NEW CULTURE

The term "corporate culture" is overused these days. But in a turnaround, culture is vital. If a turnaround is necessary, the previous organization's culture does not prohibit major problems. Indeed, the culture or lack of culture may have caused the problems. The turnaround leader must articulate a new set of values, recruit a management staff capable of practicing those values and help employees internalize them. Leaders should recognize that creating a corporate culture is not merely writing a few letters or having a few meetings. Persistent and constant follow through day in and day out is necessary to changing the attitudes of an employee group, management group and physicians. Along the way, if done effectively, a new corporate culture can bring an entirely new sense of "ownership" to all the individuals involved with the effective functioning of a hospital.

A final lesson learned was that the victory must be declared. If a turnaround succeeds, the hospital is back on its feet again and moving forward. If it fails, it will be bankrupt. One cannot sustain the adrenalin-pumping passion of turnaround leadership forever. In our organization, management, employees and physicians recognized the turnaround

was over. They began to relax, and the flexible attitudes of
the early turnaround days began to reharden. The turnaround leader must recognize these signs, declare victory
and move on to new goals beyond survival.

BEHIND EVERY LEADER

Behind every successful hospital turnaround lies a committed board. The board makes the first move in any turnaround by selecting its leader. Beyond that, it supports,
counsels and occasionally steps into the battle. Beloit Memorial Hospital's board found just the right balance between its corporate responsibilities and its desire to be
involved. Board leaders, particularly the two chairmen who
served during our turnaround, deserve much credit for our
hospital's success. Their wise counsel and occasional well-
placed kicks to the CEO's backside produced the desired
results, a hospital everyone is proud of today.

LEAD, LEAD, LEAD

Turnarounds are accomplished by leaders exercising the full
authority and responsibilities delegated to them by a board.
The turnaround process begins with the board in appoint-
ing a leader. The CEO is the architect and the team leader in
accomplishing the desired turnaround results. Along the
way, he or she uses symbols, decides on the timing of bold
moves and has the ability to vary management style according to the circumstances.

   More than anything else, a turnaround leader needs to
believe that anything is possible and that miracles can be
achieved. There are many hospital success stories. Beloit
Memorial Hospital is only one of them. But our success
should give hope to any hospital that believes failure and
bankruptcy is inevitable. It isn't. Any organization can be
rescued from a death spiral and then rise higher than it has
ever been before. To be part of such a turnaround is the
thrill of a lifetime.

APPENDIX A

Position Description: President and Chief Executive Officer

I. APPOINTMENT

The board of trustees shall select a president of the corporation. The president shall be the chief executive officer of the corporation with all of the authority common to the office of the president of a business corporation. The president shall have all authority and responsibility necessary to operate the corporation in all of its activities and departments, subject only to such policies as may be issued by the board of trustees. He or she shall act as the duly authorized representative of the board of trustees and the corporation in all matters in which the board has not formally designated some other person to act.

II. QUALIFICATIONS

The person appointed as president shall have completed a formal education in a graduate program in hospital or business administration in a recognized college or university, and a minimum of seven (7) years experience in a responsible administrative position in a hospital, or in the health care field.

III. ACCOUNTABILITY

The president shall report to the board of trustees, and as directed to the chairman of the board of trustees between board meetings, and to the executive committee of the board of trustees, at each meeting of those bodies.

IV. COMPENSATION

The compensation, terms and conditions of appointment and services to be rendered to the corporation, of the president, shall be established by the board of trustees and updated annually, or more frequently as deemed appropriate by the board of trustees.

V. AUTHORITY AND DUTIES

More specifically, the authority and duties of the president shall be:

A. *Board relationships and development*

1. Works closely with the board of trustees to enhance its effectiveness in meeting the needs of the corporation.
2. Informs and interests trustees in current trends, issues, problems, and activities in health care generally, in community healthcare needs at the institution, to facilitate policy making.
3. Recommends policy positions concerning legislation, government and other matters of public policy.
4. Provides comprehensive and accurate information for trustees, for their use in decision making and policy matters.
5. Assists with identifying potential board members.
6. Submits regularly to the board and its committees, periodic reports showing the professional services and financial activities of the corporation, and prepares such special reports as may be required by the board.
7. Attends all meetings of the board and its committees.
8. Interprets the meaning of these by-laws and all other regulations and policies adopted by the board as they may apply in case of uncertainty or

dispute, to have the meaning that the president has been authorized and empowered by the board to be the chief executive officer of the corporation, and the decision of the president shall govern, unless otherwise specifically overruled by the actions of the board of trustees.

B. *Planning*
   1. Participates with the board in charting the course of the corporation in response to the needs of the community.
   2. Evaluates the effects of external forces on the corporation, and integrates appropriate responses into the corporation's short and long range plans.
   3. Recommends long range plans to the board which support the corporation's statement of mission and statement of corporate goals.
   4. Completes an annual operating plan to facilitate achievement of goals established in the corporation's long-range plan.

C. *Management and professional staff*
   1. Ensures the attainment of corporation goals through the selection, development, motivation and evaluation of all corporate management and professional staff.
   2. Develops and implements plan of organization to meet the needs of the corporation.
   3. Selects, employs, controls, and discharges all management and professional staff members of the corporation.
   4. Establishes formal responsibilities and accountabilities of all members of the management and professional staff, and evaluates their performance regularly.
   5. Establishes compensation and benefits for all members of the management and professional staff.

6. Negotiates professional contracts and ensures that appropriate salary or contractual rates are developed and maintained.

D. *Human resource management*

1. Ensures the patient care and operational needs of the corporation are attained through the selection, training, motivation and evaluation of all employees of the corporation.
2. Implements appropriate staffing levels and a plan of departmentalization to facilitate effective delivery of patient care and support services.
3. Specifies personnel accountability and ensures that performance is evaluated regularly.
4. Establishes compensation and benefits consistent with board approved limitations.

E. *Quality of healthcare services*

1. Monitors the adequacy of the corporation's medical activities, appointments, reappointments and medical staff privileges, through coordination with the board, medical staff and patient care staff, the policies needed to assure quality healthcare services.
2. Creates an operating environment which facilitates the effective practice of medicine by the physician members of the medical staff.
3. Consults with leaders of the medical and dental staff concerning patient care needs and allocation of resources to effectively meet those needs.
4. Represents the board of trustees before the medical staff of Beloit Memorial Hospital.
5. Coordinates the recruitment and retention of members of the medical staff of Beloit Memorial Hospital.

F. *Allocation of resources*

1. Promotes delivery of healthcare services in a cost effective manner and consistent with maintaining of an acceptable level of quality.

2. Assures the sound fiscal operation of the corporation including developing a comprehensive annual operating budget, and implementing that budget following board approval.

3. Develops a capital equipment budget and implements that budget following board approval.

4. Plans the use and maintenance of the physical resources of the corporation.

5. Insures all corporation property against damage.

6. Supervises all business affairs of the corporation and ensures that all funds are collected and expended to maximize the operating effectiveness of the corporation.

7. Arranges contractual relationships with consultants, contractors, architects and similar professionals, in planning and developing facilities, finances and personnel programs.

8. Signs contracts, or other instruments as the authorized representative of the corporation, except in cases where execution shall have been expressly delegated by law, or the board of trustees, to some other officer or agent of the corporation.

G. *Compliance with regulations*

1. Ensures compliance with regulations governing the corporation and the rules of accrediting bodies, by continually monitoring the corporation's activities and initiating changes as required.

2. Participates in litigation against the corporation.

3. Recommends to the board of trustees the need to institute litigation.

4. Approves final settlements of all lawsuits against the corporation.

H. *Promotion of the corporation*

1. Encourages the integration of the corporation with the community by implementing effective communication and community relations programs.

2. Represents the board of trustees to the community.

3. Initiates, develops and maintains cooperative relationships with the business community and other regional healthcare providers.

4. Generates community involvement through Auxiliary, volunteer and staff programs.

5. Speaks before community and business groups about healthcare problems, and the corporation's programs to meet community healthcare needs.

I. *General*

1. Provides overall leadership and coordinates activities of all aspects of the corporation, with the objective that the entire corporation will function as an effective unit, providing the highest quality patient care and support services consistent with available resources.

2. Maintains contemporary knowledge on ideas and developments in all phases of hospital administration to the end that the president shall provide leadership for all personnel of the corporation, the board of trustees and the medical staff.

3. Promulgates and enforces all rules and regulations for the proper conduct of the corporation, and its purposes, made by and under the authority of the board of trustees. Formulates, establishes and enforces such additional procedures, rules and regulations as may be necessary to provide for the proper admission, care, safety and discharge of patients.

Position Description:
Vice President of Support Services

I. SUMMARY

Responsible for monitoring and managing the day-to-day activities of assigned departments and assisting the president in implementing Beloit Memorial Hospital's corporate objectives. Responsible for enhancing the performance and effectiveness of the organization and president.

II. REPORTING RELATIONSHIP

Reports to and is assigned responsibilities and duties by the president.

III. QUALIFICATIONS

A. Ability to successfully accomplish results defined as implementing operating objectives and all other duties and responsibilities as assigned by the president.

B. High degree of self-motivation and ability to work comfortably and effectively in a tightly structured management environment.

C. Completed action and follow through ability on all assigned projects and responsibilities.

D. Excellent perceptual and communication skills.

E. Minimum of five years progressively responsible management experience.

F. Bachelor's degree in business or related technical field. Master's degree in business, hospital administration or related technical field desirable.

IV. SUPERVISES

A. Department director staff, consistent with the current Beloit Memorial Hospital table of organization.

B. Continuously evaluates performance of department director staff with periodic reports to the president and annual written performance evaluations. Recommends salary changes for department director staff to the president.

V. REPORTING

A. Weekly staff meetings with president for reporting of status of projects, assignments and assigned departments.

B. Quarterly reports on the status of assigned annual operating objectives.

C. Continuous reporting of formal and informal information to the president which has impact on the hospital, community, medical staff or members of the hospital staff.

D. Special reports as assigned by the president.

VI. DUTIES AND RESPONSIBILITIES

A. *Departmental operations*
   1. Oversees day-to-day activities of assigned departments and implements operating objectives in

conjunction with department directors. Implements decisions and assignments of the president. Makes decisions concerning day-to-day operating activities within established parameters and monitors departmental conformance to hospital policies, systems and procedures.

2. Continuously monitors department operating systems, policies, procedures and activities to facilitate the hospital in meeting its overall obligations to patients, medical staff and personnel.

3. Responsible for identifying policy and procedure improvements which will improve the operating effectiveness of assigned departments and for recommending policy and procedure updates to implement identified improvements.

B. *Financial responsibilities*

1. Responsible for ensuring that assigned departments are managed within established operating budget limits unless specific exceptions are made by the president.

2. Responsible for ensuring that capital equipment is acquired for assigned departments in accordance with approved capital budget.

C. *Planning*

1. Prepares annual operating plan for assigned departments.

2. In conjunction with the president and chief financial officer, assists in development of the annual operating budget and annual capital budget for each assigned department.

3. Ad hoc planning assignments for the president.

D. *Staff development*

1. Responsible for the development of strategies to improve the performance, effectiveness and morale of assigned department directors.

2. Responsible for making recommendations for

promotion, demotion or termination of assigned department director staff to facilitate accomplishing overall objectives of the Hospital.

E. *Recruitment*
   1. Responsible for recruiting members of the department director staff as vacancies occur, and recommending final candidate for hiring to the president.
   2. Coordination of the recruitment of supervisory level people in assigned departments and for approving department director's selection.

F. *Inter-departmental coordination*
   Responsible for the effective inter-department coordination between assigned departments and departments responsible to other administrative directors. Responsible for coordinating inter-departmental committees and task forces as assigned by the president.

G. *Regulatory compliance*
   Responsible for ensuring that assigned departments comply with all accreditation requirements and local, state and federal licensing and operating requirements.

H. *Meetings and committee assignments*
   Represents president at internal and external meetings, committees, functions, etc. as assigned.

I. *Additional responsibilities*
   Other ad hoc staff assignments for president as requested.

APPENDIX C

Position Description: Director of Human Resources

I. SUMMARY

The position is responsible and accountable for the design, development, maintenance and implementation of all personnel programs, policies and procedures necessary to:

A. Secure and retain qualified personnel at all levels in the organization.

B. Maintain competitive wage, salary and benefit programs.

C. Control personnel expenses consistent with the Beloit Memorial Hospital's annual operating budget.

D. Promote productive work habits and maintenance of an atmosphere free of labor disharmony.

E. Assure compliance with state and federal laws which relate to the personnel function.

F. Promote managerial effectiveness of first-line supervisors, department managers and members of the administrative staff through competent consultation on personnel matters.

G. Assure compliance with current union contracts

II. REPORTING RELATIONSHIPS
Position reports to and is assigned responsibilities and duties by the president.

III. SUPERVISES

A. Supervises all human resources department employees, consistent with current hospital table of organization.

B. Exercises staff responsibility on all human resource matters.

IV. SKILLS, KNOWLEDGE AND ABILITIES

A. Minimum of five years personnel department experience and three years supervisory level experience is necessary.

B. Experience with negotiating and administering union contracts is necessary.

C. Bachelor's degree in personnel management or related field is necessary.

D. Master's degree in management-related discipline is desirable.

E. Ability to successfully accomplish results defined as implementing corporate and human resources department operating objectives and all other duties assigned by the president.

F. High degree of self-motivation, personal organization, institutional commitment and creativity.

G. Excellent written and oral communication skills, and ability to relate well to all staff levels.

V. CHARACTERISTIC DUTIES AND RESPONSIBILITIES

A. *Department operations*
1. Maintain employee records.
2. Administer benefit system.
3. Fill open positions.
4. Monitor position control program.
5. Prepare periodic personnel data reports.
6. Monitor and assess other operational systems.

B. *Planning*
1. Prepare annual operating plan and evaluation of the human resources department to include major trends and staff issue analysis.
2. Develop and implement annual operating objectives for the department.
3. Assist the finance department in preparing the hospital annual operating budget.
4. Prepare manpower needs forecast to cover a three-year period, updated annually.
5. Prepare three-year plan for employee benefits improvements, updated annually.
6. Prepare other reports as directed by the president.

C. *Staff concerns and issues*
1. Monitor and assess employee and management staff concerns and issues.
2. Communicate issues continuously to the president for followup as appropriate.

D. *Staff retention*
Develop and implement, through department managers, strategies to retain qualified and competent employees.

E. *Control and audit*
Develop and implement comprehensive audit programs to ensure effective compliance with all hospital personnel policies and procedures.

F. *Consultation to management staff*
    Provide competent consultation to first-line supervisors, department managers and administrative staff on employee discipline, evaluations, problem solving and other personnel matters to enhance the effectiveness of the line management staff.

G. *Policy formulation and implementation*
    Develop and assist in the implementation of all hospital personnel policies.

H. *Financial controls*
    1. Monitor of hospital personnel expenses, to include overtime expenses, authorized staff levels, sick and absenteeism utilization and tardiness in order to facilitate optimal use of hospital financial resources.
    2. Prepare exception reports to the appropriate management staff as necessary to ensure control is maintained over personnel expenses.

I. *Wage and salary administration*
    1. Monitor, assess and maintain a competitive wage and salary program and make recommendations for change in wage, salary and benefit programs where appropriate.
    2. Evaluate hospital positions in order to maintain internal wage and salary consistency between departments.

J. *Regulatory and legal issues*
    1. Maintain current knowledge on all state, federal, state health code and JCAH requirements regarding personnel issues.
    2. Identify problem areas and communicate them to the president for followup.

K. *Program evaluation and consultation*
    Evaluate personnel and organizational programs for the vice presidents and president as requested.

L. *Contract negotiations*
Lead hospital's union contract negotiating team, including strategy development and bargaining table negotiations.

M. *Contract maintenance*
Oversee union contract, including grievance procedures and wage and benefit administration.

N. *Reporting*
1. Brief the president weekly on the status of personnel issues and problems.
2. Report and convey informed opinions and observations to keep the department managers, vice presidents and president apprised of all issues which have impact on the hospital, employees or community.
3. Prepare monthly personnel operations summary, with analysis of current employee issues and trends.
4. Prepare other reports, as assigned by the president.

O. *Committee assignments*
1. Member of safety committee.
2. Advisor to social committee.
3. Other committees as assigned by the president.

P. *Ad hoc assignments*
1. Represent hospital at internal and external meetings, functions, etc., as assigned by the president.
2. Ad hoc staff assignments for the president as requested.

Long-Range Plan Questions

BOARD OF TRUSTEES QUESTIONS

1. *Hospital strengths* - What are the hospital's three greatest strengths?

2. *Hospital weaknesses* - What are the hospital's three greatest weaknesses?

3. *Community* - What changes do you project for the greater Beloit community in terms of population, employment and image between now and 1990?

4. *Medical needs* - What are the greatest medical needs in the greater Beloit community?

5. *Service and facility needs* - What medical services or facilities would you most like to see developed in Beloit between now and 1990?

6. *1990 goal* - What is the single greatest issue or opportunity which needs to be addressed to position Beloit Memorial Hospital as the best community hospital in the United States?

7. *Performance measurement* - What are the best objective indicators to measure the hospital's long-range performance?

8. *Other insights* - What other comments or insights would you like to make as part of our long-range plan update?

MEDICAL STAFF QUESTIONS

1. *Hospital Strengths* - What are the hospital's three greatest strengths?

2. *Hospital Weaknesses* - What are the hospital's three greatest weaknesses?

3. *Hospital-Based Physicians* - Rate the overall quality and service of hospital-based physicians:

	Excellent		Average		Poor
A. Emergency Medicine	1	2	3	4	5
B. Pathology	1	2	3	4	5
C. Radiology	1	2	3	4	5
D. Anesthesiology	1	2	3	4	5

4. *Medical strengths* - What are our greatest physician strengths?

5. *Medical weaknesses* - What are our greatest physician weaknesses?

6. *Service and facility needs* - What new medical services or new hospital facilities would you most like to see developed between now and 1990?

7. *Equipment* - What major (over $100,000) new medical equipment would you most like to see purchased between now and 1990?

8. *Other insights* - What other comments or insights would you like to offer as part of our long-range plan update?

COMMUNITY LEADER QUESTIONS

1. *Hospital strengths* - What are the hospital's greatest strengths?

2. *Hospital weaknesses* - What are the hospital's greatest weaknesses?

3. *Community* - What changes do you project for the greater Beloit community in terms of population, employment and image between now and 1990?

4. *Physician image* - What is the overall image of physicians practicing in Beloit?

5. *Physician needs* - What are the greatest physician needs in the greater Beloit community?

6. *Service and facility needs* - What medical services or facilities would you most like to see developed in Beloit between now and 1990?

7. *Out-migration* - What is the single most important change or improvement necessary to reduce the number of Beloit residents seeking medical care outside the community?

8. *Other insights* - What other comments or insights would you like made as part of our long-range plan update?

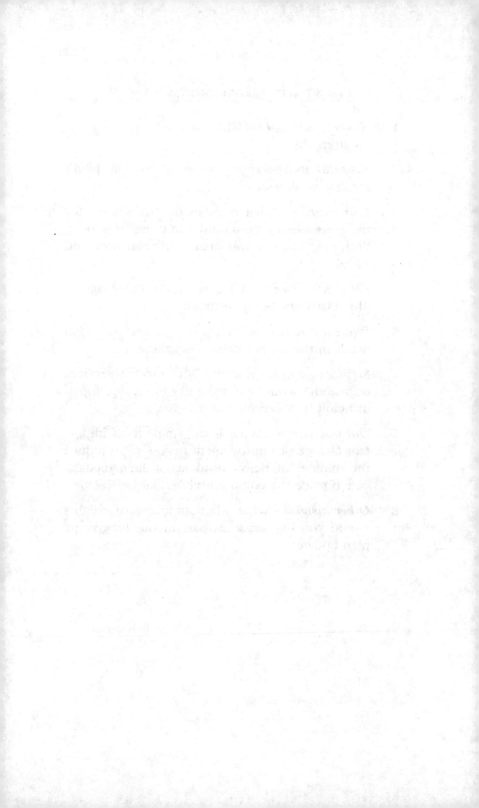

Index

A

Aiken, George, Senator, 199
American Hospital Association
    Data Center, ix–x
American Hospital Association
    Monitrend studies, 32–33
Automated cart delivery
    systems, 56–57

B

Beloit Memorial Hospital, 2–4,
    10–11, 17
    advertising for, 132–34,
        139–51, 176
    board of trustees of, 10–11,
        197–98, 222
    day surgery at, 160–61, 170,
        185
    emergency medical services
        at, 153–55, 188–89, 191–92
    equipment and, 161–63,
        170–71
    inpatient activity at, 3, 91
    management size and, 20–21,
        22–27, 54–56, 193–94
    nursing staff of, 22, 26, 33

physician specialists and,
        157–60
    Plan 1990 for, 201–09
    rate freeze at, 183–84
    referrals and, 156–57, 167–68
    senior citizens and, 186
    Sports Medicine Center at,
        185–86
    staff reductions at, 36–38
    stategies for, 98–102, 179–80
    subcontracting services for,
        187–188
    volunteers at, 82, 84
Britton, Gregory, 107–08
Business cards, 137–38

C

Carlzon, Jan, 120
Chioutsis, John, 108–09
Columbus Medical Center
    (Chicago), 70
Corporate culture, 117–26,
    221–22

E

Earl, Anthony, Governor, 157

Index

Employee issues, 71–75, 95–96,
195–96

G

General Electric, 88
Gerhardt, Vanetta, 106

H

Hospital
board of trustees, 11–12,
15–17, 219–20
chief executive officer of,
10–11, 15–17, 86–88,
198–99, 220, 223–28
director of human resources
for, 233–37
lobbies, 81–83, 89–90
patient day statistics for, 3
symbols and, 79–90
turnaround warning signs for,
1–2
vice president of support
services for, 229–32
See also management changes,
physician issues
Hospital service expenses, 51,
57–58
accounting and, 52
dues and network fees as, 53
liquid oxygen and, 52
maintenance contracts and,
53–54
rental costs and, 52–53
Hospital staff reductions, 29,
32–34, 40–41
communicating about, 30
media and, 38–39
physicians and, 39–40
strategy for, 35–36
unions and, 31–32
See also Beloit Memorial
Hospital

J

Jones, Reginald, 88

M

Management changes, 12–13,
19–20, 75–77, 105–15
See also Beloit Memorial
Hospital
Market research, 63–68, 91–94,
175–78
Media, 89
hospital advertising and, 142
Moosebrugger, Mary, 66–67
Morgan, John, 106

O

Outplacement counseling, 27,
41

P

Patient complaints, 129–32
Patient welcome cards, 127–29
Physician focus groups, 94
Physician issues, 13–14, 70–71,
85–86, 168–70, 196–97
Pollard, William H., M.D.,
Ambulatory Surgery Unit, 161
Purvis, George, 70

Q

Quigley Associates, 112

R

Rynne Marketing Group, 65, 99

S

SWOT assessment, 96–98